Eosinophils and Their Role in Human Health and Disease

Edited by Seyyed Shamsadin Athari, Entezar Mehrabi Nasab and Luis Rodrigo

Published in London, United Kingdom

Eosinophils and Their Role in Human Health and Disease
http://dx.doi.org/10.5772/intechopen.1001704
Edited by Seyyed Shamsadin Athari, Entezar Mehrabi Nasab and Luis Rodrigo

Contributors
Alberto Garcia-Garcia, Ashley A. Seymour, Asuman Akkaya Fırat, Aychin I. Hasanova, Barbara Saenz-Ibarra, Brian W.P. Seymour, Emin Kh. Verdiyev, Ferid V. Guliyev, Fidan N. Gasimova, Gulustan H. Babayeva, Gulustan H. Babayeva, Gulzar R. Aliyeva, Gunay V. Asadova, Hikmet I. Ibrahimli, Irada M. Akhundova, Jamal S. Musayev, Jeyhun M. Ismayilzada, Konul M. Kerimova, Namig O. Isgandarov, Nargiz E. Afandiyeva, Nargiz N. Huseynova, Natavan A. Farajova, Natavan R. Ismailova, Odewusi Odeyinka Olufunsho, Omon Emmanuel Akokhamen, Patricia M. Gilford, Rafail H. Hasanov, Rafiq I. Bayramov, Rashad A. Hasanov, Rosario Medellin-Vallejo, Sadagat S. Sultanova, Susana Jiménez-Contreras, Tunzala A. Maharramova, Umud R. Mahmudov, Zulfu Sh. Gadimova

First published in London, United Kingdom, 2024 by IntechOpen
IntechOpen is the global imprint of INTECHOPEN LIMITED, registered in England and Wales, registration number: 11086078, 167-169 Great Portland Street, London, W1W 5PF, United Kingdom

British Library Cataloguing-in-Publication Data
A catalogue record for this book is available from the British Library

Additional hard and PDF copies can be obtained from orders@intechopen.com

Eosinophils and Their Role in Human Health and Disease
Edited by Seyyed Shamsadin Athari, Entezar Mehrabi Nasab and Luis Rodrigo
p. cm.
Print ISBN 978-0-85466-731-4
Online ISBN 978-0-85466-730-7
eBook (PDF) ISBN 978-0-85466-732-1

For EU product safety concerns:
IN TECH d.o.o., Prolaz Marije Krucifikse Kozulić 3, 51000 Rijeka, Croatia,
info@intechopen.com or visit our website at intechopen.com.

Meet the editors

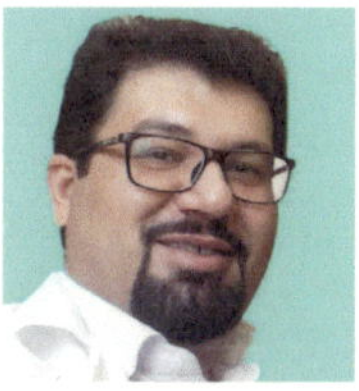

Dr. Seyyed Shamsadin Athari is an assistant professor of immunology in the Department of Immunology, School of Medicine, Zanjan University of Medical Sciences, Zanjan, Iran, and has an allergy and asthma toxicology postdoctorate and an asthma management and controlling network fellowship. He published more than 250 manuscripts in international journals in the fields of immunology, allergy, and asthma and has written more than 35 books. He is also on the editorial board of more than 90 international journals in medical sciences, has inventions in medical sciences, and has recorded gene sequences in a gene bank. Dr. Athari has been invited as a top speaker in more than 50 international congresses and symposiums and has received scientific awards from different scientific societies as a young top researcher and young scientist.

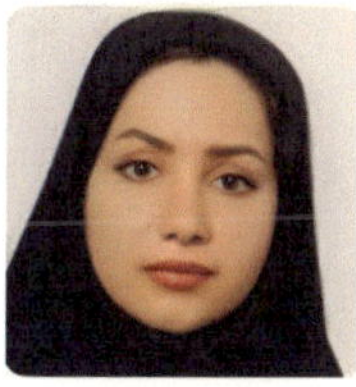

Dr. Entezar Mehrabi Nasab, MD, is a cardiologist specializing in cardiovascular diseases and holds a fellowship in interventional clinical electrophysiology, and completed her residency and fellowship at the Tehran Heart Center, Tehran University of Medical Sciences, Iran. She has published more than 40 scientific articles in international journals. She has been an invited speaker at more than 30 international congresses. Dr. Mehrabi Nasab has received awards from different scientific societies.

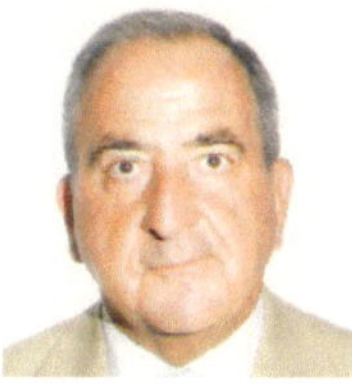

Luis Rodrigo has been a full professor of medicine at the University of Oviedo (Spain) since 2010 and an emeritus professor since 2014. He has been a specialist in gastroenterology since 1972, achieving his Ph.D. in 1975 and being appointed as titular professor in medicine at the University of Oviedo in 1983. He has been head of the Gastroenterology Service of HUCA in Oviedo since 1975. He is the author of 14 books on the treatment of gastroenterological and other digestive and liver diseases, has contributed 58 chapters to other medical books, and is the main author or coauthor of 459 scientific papers in English and another 282 in Spanish.

Contents

Preface

Eosinophils are one of the main immune system cells that play a homeostatic role in the body and immune responses. The eosinophil cell is involved in combating parasitic, viral, and bacterial infections and certain cancers and has pathologic roles in diseases including allergy, asthma, chronic rhino-sinusitis with nasal polyps, eosinophilic gastrointestinal disorders, and hyper-eosinophilic syndromes. The human eosinophil typically comprises about 1–5% of all circulating WBCs, has long been felt to favorably impact innate mucosal immunity, and has also been incriminated in disease pathophysiology. Eosinophils, like other circulating lymphocytes, are developed from the multipotent hematopoietic stem cells in bone marrow, and eosinophil-committed progenitors are terminally differentiated into mature eosinophils in the presence of several growth factors (such as cytokines) and transcription factors. Moreover, eosinophils also interact with other WBCs and regulate their functions, ranging from their role in the T-cell selection to enhancing the macrophages' ability to phagocytize apoptotic thymic cells. When exposed to inflammatory signals, eosinophils enter inflamed tissues, where they function as main mediators of effector function and innate immunity, as well as participate in the adaptive immune responses.

In this book, we present eosinophil-related mechanisms that are involved in the pathophysiology of diseases and focus on the related problems. We review the molecular mechanisms involved in control of eosinophil reactions. Furthermore, we discuss the views on the role of eosinophils in innate and adaptive immunity and in disease processes and related disorders. We hope this book will be applicable and useful for all researchers, clinicians, paraclinics, drug designers, and other related biomedical scientists.

Dr. Seyyed Shamsadin Athari
Zanjan University of Medical Sciences,
Zanjan, Iran

Dr. Entezar Mehrabi Nasab
Tehran University of Medical Sciences,
Tehran, Iran

Dr. Luis Rodrigo
University of Oviedo,
Oviedo, Spain,

Hospital Universitario Central de Asturias,
Oviedo, Spain

Chapter 1

Eosinophilic Esophagitis: Update and Review

Susana Jiménez-Contreras and Alberto Garcia-Garcia

Abstract

Eosinophilic esophagitis (EoE) is a chronic immune-mediated clinicopathological condition characterized by symptoms of esophageal dysfunction (dysphagia and food impaction) along with esophageal biopsies showing an eosinophilic infiltrate in the mucosa of 15 or more eosinophils per 0.3 mm^3 field, excluding other causes of esophageal eosinophilia. Its prevalence has tripled in the last 10 years. This increase cannot solely be attributed to the rise in gastroscopies performed or greater awareness of the disease among health professionals. It is more common in men, particularly in Western countries, and can be associated with other allergic diseases such as asthma, allergic rhinitis, or atopic dermatitis. Diagnosis is based on the histological examination of esophageal biopsies. Various treatments are available, including proton pump inhibitors, corticosteroids, empiric exclusion diets, or biological drugs. Disease progression can lead to esophageal fibrosis and strictures that may necessitate treatment with endoscopic dilation.

Keywords: eosinophilic esophagitis, dysphagia, eosinophil, food impaction, atopy, food allergy, elimination diet

1. Introduction

Eosinophilic esophagitis (EoE) was first described in 1993 by Attwood [1] and 1 year later by Straumann [2] as an entity with its own clinical and histological characteristics. Previously, some authors interpreted the presence of eosinophils in the esophageal mucosa as a sign of GERD. In 1995 Kelly et al. described a series of 23 children with GERD refractory to medical and surgical treatment who responded to an elemental diet [3]. The first consensus guideline on EoE was published in 2007 [4]. Since then, interest in EoE has increased from being considered a rare entity to becoming a common diagnosis. It is currently the second cause of esophageal inflammation after gastroesophageal reflux disease (GERD) and the most common cause of dysphagia and food impaction in children and young adults [5–7].

EoE is associated with the Th2 lymphocyte-mediated inflammatory response, and is considered a form of food allergy, and shares mechanisms of action with atopic diseases such as asthma or atopic dermatitis. In its pathogenesis, the role of eotaxins and interleukins (IL) 13 and 5 stands out.

The most common clinical presentation at diagnosis is dysphagia and food impaction. Diagnosis should be histological, with the most characteristic feature being the presence of an inflammatory infiltrate of eosinophils, which by definition should be greater than 15 eosinophils per field of 0.3 mm^3. There are various effective treatments for EoE, ranging from proton pump inhibitors (PPIs), elimination diets, topical corticosteroids, and more recently, biologic drugs. The most frequent complication is esophageal stricture, caused by subepithelial fibrosis secondary to chronic inflammation, and its most effective treatment is endoscopic dilation, with or without topical corticosteroids.

2. Definition

EoE is a defined as a chronic type 2-associated inflammatory disease, immune or antigen driven, characterized by predominant eosinophilic inflammation of the esophagus (greater than or equal to 15 eosinophils per 0.3 mm^3 field). Clinically, it is characterized by symptoms related to esophageal dysfunction, with dysphagia and esophageal dysfunction being its predominant symptoms. Years ago, it was necessary to exclude GERD before establishing a diagnosis of EoE. But currently, infiltration by eosinophils in the esophageal epithelium after 2 months of treatment with PPIs is no longer a diagnostic criterion to exclude EoE, but PPIs have become part of the treatment of EoE [8]. This is because it was observed that patients with dysphagia and food impactions who responded to PPIs exhibited the same phenotypic, molecular, and therapeutic characteristics as those who did not respond [9, 10].

There are other entities that present with esophageal eosinophilia and that must be ruled out before establishing a diagnosis of EoE, such as Crohn's disease, collagen vascular disease, hypereosinophilic syndrome, GERD and esophagitis induced by drugs or infections.

3. Epidemiology

Cases of EoE have been described throughout the world although epidemiological studies have been published in North America, Australia, and Europe. The studies are heterogeneous in terms of the methodology used (case series, randomized clinical trials, case-control studies...) as well as the definitions of EoE used, since this has been modified over the years. Different cut-off points regarding the number of eosinophils are used and the oldest studies exclude EoE that responds to treatment with PPIs as it was considered a different entity.

Incidence rate of EoE appears to be increasing according to the latest published studies. The annual incidence at the Mayo Clinic went from 0.35 cases per 100,000 person-years between 1991 and 1995 to 9.45 cases per 100,000 person-years between 2001 and 2005 [6]. Similarly, other European studies have shown an increase in incidence between 10 and 20 times in less than 20 years [11, 12]. Possible causes would be greater awareness of this entity among gastroenterologists, as well as greater access to endoscopy. But studies suggest that the increase in the incidence rate is due not only to an increase in diagnosis, but also to an actual increase in the disease.

As a result of this increase in incidence, added to the fact that patients are usually diagnosed at an early age and that it does not reduce their life expectancy, the prevalence of EoE has also increased in recent years. Thus, the prevalence has gone from 42.96 cases per 100,000 inhabitants published in 2004 in the United States to current rates between 81 and 100 cases per 100,000 inhabitants published as of 2016 [13–15].

More recent studies have described prevalence above 100 cases per 100,000 inhabitants in both children and adults [14, 15].

The hygiene theory is one of the reasons that would explain the enormous increase in the prevalence of EoE. Like EoE, other diseases related to more sterile environments, especially during childhood, such as atopic dermatitis, asthma, rhinitis, inflammatory bowel disease or food allergies, have also experienced a notable increase in their prevalence in the last decades. The sterile environment limits the exposure of the immune system to antigenic stimuli, hindering its maturation and promoting hyperreactivity against self or external antigens [16]. It is unknown why foods such as milk, eggs, wheat, or legumes, so common in our diet for thousands of years, are the main triggers for this disease.

Since the definition of EoE changed in 2017–2018 [8, 17], and the response to PPIs transitioned from being a diagnostic criterion to a treatment for the disease, a significant number of patients were included in prevalence and incidence rates. Finally, increased awareness and knowledge among healthcare professionals (not only gastroenterologists) about the disease have allowed for a greater number of diagnoses, both in patients with recent clinical onset and those with long-standing compatible symptoms who had not yet been diagnosed [7].

Different risk factors have been associated with the development of EoE: living in geographical areas with colder temperatures and higher humidity, male sex, Caucasian race, older children and age between 30 and 45 years in adults, atopy, family history of EoE (possible common genetic changes although a shared environmental environment also seems necessary), breastfeeding, and admission to neonatal ICU [7]. The role of aeroallergens and seasonality, extensively studied in EoE, was questioned in a systematic review and meta-analysis published in 2015 with 16,846 patients from 18 studies [18].

4. Etiopathogenesis

Eosinophils are granulocytes produced by the bone marrow related to the immune response to parasitic infections and allergic phenomena. Under normal conditions, the esophageal mucosa does not contain any eosinophils, unlike other organs of the digestive system. Interleukin 5 (IL-5) is considered the main inducer of their expansion and subsequent release into the bloodstream [19] and was one of the first targets in the search for possible treatments for EoE [20]. Once in the blood, eosinophils are recruited by the esophagus through mediators produced by the inflamed tissue, although this mechanism is not well understood yet. Some of the proposed mechanisms studied as potential therapeutic targets include: increased expression of the DD chemokine receptor cCR3 common for eotaxins [21], intercellular adhesion molecule (ICAM)-1 [22], integrin CD11c, prostaglandin D2 receptor CRTH2 [22, 23], and mRNA FLOXP3 [23].

The intestinal epithelium has emerged as a fundamental defense mechanism in maintaining intestinal homeostasis, serving both as a barrier function and mediating between bacteria and the immune system [24, 25]. Esophageal epithelial cells express molecules of the major histocompatibility complex (MHC) class II acting as antigen-presenting cells [21, 23].

In EoE, eosinophils are distributed in an ascending gradient from the superficial layers, in contact with ingested antigens, to the deeper layers [26]. Additionally, they cluster to form microabscesses in the superficial strata [27, 28].

In active EoE, alterations have been demonstrated at different levels in its epithelial barrier: in tight junctions with alteration of some of their components (claudin-1, claudin-4, occludin or proteins of the occludin-1 zonula) [29], in structural proteins responsible for maintaining mucosal integrity (such as E-cadherin, involucrin, or filaggrin) [30, 31], and in the expression of the cytoskeletal protein synaptopodin [32]. All these changes have been related to the depletion of the serine protease inhibitor, kazal type (SPINK) 7, absent in the epithelium of patients with active EoE, contrary to what happens with healthy controls [33]. As a consequence, there is an increase in epithelial permeability, with dilated intercellular spaces allowing the passage of antigens, demonstrated by the overexpression of epithelial antimicrobial peptides and the upregulation of bacterial pattern recognition Toll-like [29, 34].

Thymic stromal lymphopoietin (TSLP), a cytokine closely related to immune-mediated processes such as asthma, atopic dermatitis, inflammatory bowel disease, and EoE, is mainly produced in the esophageal epithelium by epithelial cells, fibroblasts, and other stromal cells. Its induction mechanism is unknown, but it is highly relevant in the activation of antigen-presenting cells, which promote the maturation of T lymphocytes into Th2 cells. Activated Th2 cells secrete cytokines such as IL-13, a key cytokine in EoE. In EoE, IL-13 promotes epithelial dysfunction by dysregulating genes related to the epithelial barrier (CAPN14), reducing proteins like desmoglein-1, inhibiting the expression of filaggrin and involucrin, and altering the expression pattern of TJ-associated proteins [35].

Since its description in 1993, EoE has been associated with atopy. Both patients and their family members suffer more frequently than the general population from diseases such as asthma, allergic rhinitis, atopic dermatitis, drug hypersensitivity, eosinophilia, or elevated levels of IgE in serum [36]. IgE-mediated food allergies are also more common [37]. This significant increase in immune-mediated diseases has been partially justified by the hygiene hypothesis, according to which reduced exposure to allergens during childhood produces changes in the microbiota that condition an altered response of T lymphocytes [38]. In this sense, invariant natural killer T (iNKT) cells, which are stimulated by glycolipid antigens through class I MHC proteins and are related to phenomena of immunotolerance, have been shown to play an essential role in the pathophysiology of EoE. iNKT cells are capable of inducing EoE in animal models [39, 40], are more numerous in the epithelium of patients with EoE compared to healthy controls [41], and furthermore, they normalize after removing allergens from the diet.

Mast cells, mesenchymal cells derived from bone marrow myeloid cells, are increased in patients with active EoE and decrease, like eosinophils, after effective treatment [35]. Mast cell infiltration density has been proposed as a mechanism to differentiate EoE from GERD [42, 43].

In EoE, genetic susceptibility has been demonstrated, which, along with environmental factors and the immune system of each patient, are responsible for the development of the disease. The main gene identified in patients with EoE is eotaxin-3/CCL26, with a 53-fold higher risk than controls. The TSLP receptor and its ligand have been identified in children with EoE [44]. Some single nucleotide polymorphisms (SNPs) have also been identified as risk factors for the disease (genes CCL26, TGFβ and its LRRC32 protein, FLG, TSLP, DSG1, CRLF2, and TLR3) [35]. The predominance of EoE in males has been related to genetic alterations of the sex chromosomes. Thus, mutations in two chains of the IL-13 receptor gene located on the X chromosome, not corrected by the Y chromosome in males, and more recently, an SNP in the gene encoding the TSLP receptor are the most associated with male predominance in EoE [45].

As a result of chronic esophageal inflammation, subepithelial fibrosis occurs, which is common to other processes with eosinophilic inflammatory infiltrates. This fibrosis occurs as a consequence of untreated or inadequately treated inflammation and has been described in children, adults, and animal models, although it does not occur in all cases. Clinically, fibrosis leads to dysmotility, esophageal rigidity, progressive dysphagia, food impaction, and ultimately, stenosis [35]. The main factor associated with progression to fibrosis is transforming growth factor (TGF)-β1, the same factor described for asthma [46].

5. Clinical features

Symptomatology differs between children and adults. Children may present with a wide variety of non-specific symptoms such as abdominal pain, nausea and vomiting, and failure to thrive. Though it is still being characterized, feeding dysfunction is becoming more often acknowledged as an EoE manifestation. It comprises the inability to establish typical eating behaviors (such as not progressing past liquids or soft foods) and the adoption of coping mechanisms (such as eating slowly, chewing food excessively, or refusing to eat solids after having previously eaten them) [47].

In contrast, teenagers and adults are more likely to present with dysphagia, episodes of food impaction and non-swallowing associated chest pain. Dysphagia to solid foods is the most common symptom (70–80%). EoE is discovered in up to 15% of individuals undergoing endoscopic evaluation for dysphagia [6]. As many as 54% of patients have a history of food impaction [48]. Heartburn, especially with the ingestion of alcohol, occurs in 30% of adult patients. Rarely, eosinophilic esophagitis may manifest with spontaneous rupture of the esophagus from forceful retching (Boerhaave's syndrome) after food impaction [49, 50].

The natural history of the disease in untreated patients progresses from the initial inflammatory pattern, characterized by eosinophilic infiltration as the main histological change, to structural changes with subepithelial fibrosis leading to dysmotility, esophageal rigidity, progressive dysphagia, food impaction, and ultimately, the formation of strictures [7]. The fibrostenotic pattern is uncommon, and although we can find it in both children and adults, the risk of its occurrence doubles with each decade of disease progression without proper diagnosis and treatment [51–53].

6. Diagnosis

Diagnosis requires the presence of symptoms related to esophageal dysfunction, the presence of an eosinophilic infiltrate in esophageal biopsies and the exclusion of other causes that could lead to both situations [8].

6.1 Endoscopic features

The most frequent endoscopic observations include strictures (21%), esophageal rings (44%), white spots indicating eosinophilic exudates (27%), and linear furrows (48%). The estimated frequency of each endoscopic feature according to a meta-analysis comparing 4678 patients with EoE and 2742 controls is shown in parentheses [54]. There is a validated endoscopic scoring system (EREFS) that evaluates the presence of these signs and may be useful in clinical trials [55].

6.2 Histology

Histological diagnosis of EoE is dependent on eosinophilic infiltration of the squamous epithelium. The vast majority of patients have at least 15 eosinophils per high power field (peak value) in at least one biopsy specimen. This value is thought to approach a sensitivity of 100% and specificity of 96% [8]. Biopsies should be taken from both the distal and proximal esophagus. Different studies have evaluated the number of biopsies necessary for diagnosis. At least six biopsies should be taken from different locations, focusing on areas with endoscopic mucosal abnormalities, mainly white exudates and longitudinal furrows, which are associated with higher peak eosinophil counts [17]. In turn, biopsies of the duodenum and gastric antrum should be taken to rule out eosinophilic gastroenteritis whenever suspected, as its presence may influence treatment.

Other histologic findings suggestive but not specific for EoE include eosinophil microabscesses, eosinophil surface layering, sheets of eosinophils, extracellular eosinophil granules, subepithelial and lamina propria fibrosis and inflammation, basal zone hyperplasia, papillary lengthening and increased numbers of mast cells, B cells, and IgE-bearing cells. There is an EoE-specific histologic scoring system (EoEHSS), validated *in situ*, that provides a standardized method for evaluating esophageal biopsies for features in addition to the maximum eosinophil count [56].

6.3 Radiology

Barium studies can help describe anatomic abnormalities and provide information on the length and width of strictures, but they are not sensitive enough to diagnose EoE [57]. Barium tests can also be used to evaluate luminal narrowing that is not visible during endoscopy. According to two recent investigations, esophageal narrowing was not detected during endoscopy in 71% of adults and 55% of children with eosinophilic esophagitis, but it was present during esophagography [58].

6.4 Laboratory tests

In some patients we can observe elevated IgE levels or peripheral eosinophilia, although this is usually mild.

6.5 Other diagnostic tests

Different tests have been evaluated for the diagnosis of EoE such as functional lumen imaging probe, endoscopic ultrasound, impedance planimetry to measure esophageal pressures and distensibility, mucosal impedance contour analysis that evaluates esophageal mucosal integrity, esophageal manometry, and endoscopic confocal laser microscopy. However, they are not routinely used and more studies are needed to standardize their use.

7. Treatment

Treatments for eosinophilic esophagitis vary widely in effectiveness. To date, it has not been demonstrated that combining multiple treatments is more effective than monotherapy. Additionally, combining multiple treatments can lead to errors in result interpretation and poor reproducibility of the trials [59].

We must consider that since symptoms do not correlate with histological alterations, particularly with the density of eosinophilic epithelial infiltration, after each treatment initiation or change, we should perform an endoscopy with biopsy sampling in a recommended period of 8 to 12 weeks. When implementing an empiric food elimination diet, endoscopic evaluations are conducted between 6 and 12 weeks after initiating the diet and after introducing each new food.

Regardless of the treatment that achieves disease remission, the rate of clinical and histological relapse after its withdrawal is very high, so maintenance therapy is recommended [50].

7.1 Dietary management

7.1.1 Elemental diet

The patient receives an amino acid-based formula (elemental), which eliminates all potential food allergens. This is the most effective method, able to induce histological remission in 90.8% (95%CI: 84.7–95.5%) of EoE patients of all ages, but it is difficult to follow, especially for adults, so it is rarely used [60].

7.1.2 Testing-directed elimination diet

It is based on the elimination of foods with positive results to skin prick testing and atopy patch testing. In addition, cow's milk should be eliminated due to its low negative predictive value in these tests. These diets are in disuse due to their difficulty of implementation and the greater success of elimination diets. This appears to be because the immune mechanism by which EoE develops is not IgE-mediated, an immunoglobulin directly related to food allergies, although its role, as well as that of IgG4, is still not fully understood [35].

7.1.3 Empiric elimination diet

It is the most commonly used dietary therapy. There are two types, the six-food elimination diet (cow's milk, hen's egg, soy, wheat, peanuts/tree nuts, fish/shellfish) and the four-food elimination diet (cow's milk, hen's egg, soy +/− other legumes, and wheat). The second arose due to the difficulty in carrying out a multi-food elimination diet, resulting in a lack of adherence to the diet. Sequential reintroduction of each of the excluded foods under endoscopic and histological control allows us to identify with certainty the foods responsible for EoE in each patient [61]. In addition, subsequent data showed that fish/seafood and peanuts/nuts were infrequent triggers of EoE, and foods such as cereals, legumes, and meats were more common triggers. Most patients with an identified dietary trigger respond to cow's milk and wheat elimination (two-food elimination diet). Further data have shown that the efficacy of cow's milk elimination alone is close to that of four food elimination diet and is easier to follow. A one or two food elimination diet stepping up to a more restrictive four or six food elimination has been proposed as a clinically effective strategy for dietary management of EoE [50].

7.2 Acid suppression

Among the drugs with anti-inflammatory capacity useful in EoE, several clinical trials and prospective studies in adults and children have shown that treatment with

PPIs is able to induce histological remission of the disease in 50–57% of patients [62]. An initial treatment is recommended for 8 weeks. The recommended doses of PPIs in adults comprise omeprazole 20–40 mg twice daily or equivalent; in children, 1–2 mg/kg omeprazole or equivalent. A trend toward greater efficacy has been observed when the total dose is divided into two doses per day. After 8 weeks, the clinical, endoscopic and histological response is verified. For those patients who respond to treatment, we must continue the PPI at the lowest dose successful at controlling symptoms [63].

7.3 Topical glucocorticoids

The most studied glucocorticoids in the treatment of EoE are fluticasone and budesonide.

Fluticasone propionate is administered using a metered dose inhaler without a spacer. The medication is sprayed into the patient's mouth and then swallowed. When the drug is being administered, patients should not inhale, and they should wait 30 minutes afterward to eat or drink. The optimal dose for induction is two sprays (220 mcg each), twice a day [64] and it should last for four to 8 weeks followed by assessment of symptomatic response. The endoscopic and histologic improvement should be assessed 8–12 weeks after initiating the therapy.

Budesonide. Budesonide can be administered as an oral viscous slurry. The dose varies from 1 mg daily children under the age of 10 year and up to 2 mg twice a day in older children and adults. Budesonide suspension should be taken gradually by patients over a period of 5 to 10 minutes. Following this, they should refrain from eating or drinking for 30 minutes. Budesonide in orodispersible tablets (Jorveza®) has recently been approved for its use. The recommended daily dose is 2 mg of budesonide in the form of one 1 mg tablet in the morning and one in the evening. The usual duration of treatment for induction of remission of active EoE is 6 weeks. In patients who do not show an adequate response after 6 weeks, treatment can be extended up to a maximum of 12 weeks. The orodispersible tablet should be taken after the corresponding meal. It should never be chewed or swallowed undissolved. It should be placed on the tip of the tongue and gently pressed against the roof of the mouth, where it will dissolve. This usually takes about 2 minutes. The dissolved material should be swallowed slowly with saliva as the orodispersible tablet disintegrates. The orodispersible tablet should not be taken with liquids or food. At least 30 minutes should elapse before resuming eating, drinking or oral hygiene.

7.4 Biologics

Biologic compounds are in clinical trials targeting both eosinophils, mast cells, and the Th2 inflammatory pathway. Some of them have revealed statistical improvement in eosinophil count for EoE but only dupilumab was found to have improvement in both histology and symptoms to date and has been approved for treatment of eosinophilic esophagitis in the United States and in Europe [65].

Dupilumab, a fully human monoclonal antibody, blocks the receptor for IL-4 and IL-13, essential cytokines in the activation of type 2 inflammation. It is approved for the treatment of other conditions such as atopic dermatitis, asthma, and chronic rhinosinusitis. In EoE, compared to placebo, it achieved statistically significant clinical remission (measured using the Dysphagia Symptom Questionnaire, DSQ) as well as histological remission (defined as ≤ 6 eosinophils per 0.3 mm^3 field) [66]. The recommended dose is 300 mg weekly administered subcutaneously.

7.5 Endoscopic dilatation

Esophageal strictures occur in 10% of patients. Fibrotic rings that cause a reduction in esophageal lumen are even more prevalent [51, 67]. Some strictures or narrowing are not detectable endoscopically [58] and require barium studies or distensibility testing using EndoFLIP [68, 69]. They are more common in the distal esophagus but can occur at any location along the esophagus [70].

Endoscopic dilation is an effective and safe technique for treating esophageal strictures in patients with EoE, regardless of the dilation technique used (balloon dilation or bougie dilators). The success of dilation increases when endoscopic treatment is combined with effective anti-inflammatory therapy such as topical corticosteroids [50].

Author details

Susana Jiménez-Contreras* and Alberto Garcia-Garcia
Universitary Hospital Virgen de la Victoria, Málaga, Spain

*Address all correspondence to: susana.jc10@gmail.com

References

[1] Attwood SE, Smyrk TC, Demeester TR, Jones JB. Esophageal eosinophilia with dysphagia. A distinct clinicopathologic syndrome. Digestive Diseases and Sciences. 1993;**38**(1):109-116

[2] Straumann A, Spichtin HP, Bernoulli R, Loosli J, Vögtlin J. Idiopathic eosinophilic esophagitis: A frequently overlooked disease with typical clinical aspects and discrete endoscopic findings. Schweizerische Medizinische Wochenschrift. 1994;**124**(33):1419-1429

[3] Kelly KJ, Lazenby AJ, Rowe PC, Yardley JH, Perman JA, Sampson HA. Eosinophilic esophagitis attributed to gastroesophageal reflux: Improvement with an amino acid-based formula. Gastroenterology. 1995;**109**(5):1503-1512

[4] Furuta GT, Liacouras CA, Collins MH, Gupta SK, Justinich C, Putnam PE, et al. Eosinophilic esophagitis in children and adults: A systematic review and consensus recommendations for diagnosis and treatment. Gastroenterology. 2007;**133**(4):1342-1363

[5] Dellon ES. Epidemiology of eosinophilic esophagitis. Gastroenterology Clinics of North America. 2014;**43**(2):201-218

[6] Prasad GA, Talley NJ, Romero Y, Arora AS, Kryzer LA, Smyrk TC, et al. Prevalence and predictive factors of eosinophilic esophagitis in patients presenting with dysphagia: A prospective study. The American Journal of Gastroenterology. 2007;**102**(12):2627-2632

[7] Arias Á, Lucendo AJ. Epidemiology and risk factors for eosinophilic esophagitis: Lessons for clinicians. Expert Review of Gastroenterology & Hepatology. 2020;**14**(11):1069-1082

[8] Dellon ES, Liacouras CA, Molina-Infante J, Furuta GT, Spergel JM, Zevit N, et al. Updated international consensus diagnostic criteria for eosinophilic esophagitis: Proceedings of the AGREE conference. Gastroenterology. 2018;**155**(4):1022-1033.e10

[9] Molina-Infante J, Katzka DA. Proton-pump inhibitor-responsive esophageal eosinophilia. Current Opinion in Gastroenterology. 2014;**30**(4):428-433

[10] Wen T, Dellon ES, Moawad FJ, Furuta GT, Aceves SS, Rothenberg ME. Transcriptome analysis of proton pump inhibitor-responsive esophageal eosinophilia reveals proton pump inhibitor-reversible allergic inflammation. Journal of Allergy and Clinical Immunology [Internet]. 2015;**135**(1):187-197.e4. Available from: http://www.jacionline.org/article/S0091674914012718/fulltext [Accessed: February 5, 2024]

[11] Dellon ES, Erichsen R, Baron JA, Shaheen NJ, Vyberg M, Sorensen HT, et al. The increasing incidence and prevalence of eosinophilic oesophagitis outpaces changes in endoscopic and biopsy practice: National population-based estimates from Denmark. Alimentary Pharmacology & Therapeutics. 2015;**41**(7):662-670

[12] Hruz P, Straumann A, Bussmann C, Heer P, Simon HU, Zwahlen M, et al. Escalating incidence of eosinophilic esophagitis: A 20-year prospective, population-based study in Olten County, Switzerland. The Journal of Allergy and Clinical Immunology. 2011;**128**: 1349-1350.e5

[13] Molina-Infante J, Gonzalez-Cordero PL, Ferreira-Nossa HC, Mata-Romero P, Lucendo AJ, Arias A. Rising incidence and prevalence of adult eosinophilic esophagitis in midwestern Spain (2007-2016). United European Gastroenterology Journal. 2018;**6**(1):29-37

[14] Robson J, O'Gorman M, McClain A, Mutyala K, Davis C, Barbagelata C, et al. Incidence and prevalence of pediatric eosinophilic esophagitis in Utah based on a 5-year population-based study. Clinical Gastroenterology and Hepatology. 2019;**17**(1):107-114.e1

[15] Arias Á, Lucendo AJ. Incidence and prevalence of eosinophilic oesophagitis increase continuously in adults and children in Central Spain: A 12-year population-based study. Digestive and Liver Disease. 2019;**51**(1):55-62

[16] Straumann A, Simon HU. Eosinophilic esophagitis: Escalating epidemiology? The Journal of Allergy and Clinical Immunology. 2005;**115**:418-419

[17] Lucendo AJ, Molina-Infante J, Arias Á, von Arnim U, Bredenoord AJ, Bussmann C, et al. Guidelines on eosinophilic esophagitis: Evidence-based statements and recommendations for diagnosis and management in children and adults. United European Gastroenterology Journal. 2017;**5**(3):335-358

[18] Lucendo AJ, Arias Á, Redondo-González O, González-Cervera J. Seasonal distribution of initial diagnosis and clinical recrudescence of eosinophilic esophagitis: A systematic review and meta-analysis. Allergy. 2015;**70**(12):1640-1650

[19] Rothenberg ME. Eosinophilic gastrointestinal disorders (EGID). Journal of Allergy and Clinical Immunology [Internet]. 2004;**113**(1):11-28. Available from: https://pubmed.ncbi.nlm.nih.gov/14713902/ [Accessed: February 12, 2024]

[20] Hogan SP, Rothenberg ME. Review article: The eosinophil as a therapeutic target in gastrointestinal disease. Alimentary Pharmacology & Therapeutics. 2004;**20**(11-12):1231-1240

[21] Bullock JZ, Villanueva JM, Blanchard C, Filipovich AH, Putnam PE, Collins MH, et al. Interplay of adaptive th2 immunity with eotaxin-3/c-C chemokine receptor 3 in eosinophilic esophagitis. Journal of Pediatric Gastroenterology and Nutrition [Internet]. 2007;**45**(1):22-31. Available from: https://pubmed.ncbi.nlm.nih.gov/17592361/ [Accessed: February 12, 2024]

[22] Johnsson M, Bove M, Bergquist H, Olsson M, Fornwall S, Hassel K, et al. Distinctive blood eosinophilic phenotypes and cytokine patterns in eosinophilic esophagitis, inflammatory bowel disease and airway allergy. Journal of Innate Immunity [Internet]. 2011;**3**(6):594-604. Available from: https://pubmed.ncbi.nlm.nih.gov/21921589/ [Accessed: February 12, 2024]

[23] Lingblom C, Wallander J, Ingelsten M, Bergquist H, Bove M, Saalman R, et al. Eosinophils from eosinophilic oesophagitis patients have T cell suppressive capacity and express FOXP3. Clinical and Experimental Immunology. 2017;**187**(3):455-465

[24] Mulder DJ, Pooni A, Mak N, Hurlbut DJ, Basta S, Justinich CJ. Antigen presentation and MHC class II expression by human esophageal epithelial cells: Role in eosinophilic esophagitis. The American Journal of Pathology [Internet]. 2011;**178**(2):744-753.

Available from: https://pubmed.ncbi.nlm.nih.gov/21281807/ [Accessed: February 12, 2024]

[25] Sayej WN, Foster C, Jensen T, Chatfield S, Finck C. Expanding and characterizing esophageal epithelial cells obtained from children with eosinophilic esophagitis. Pediatric Research. 2018;**84**(2):306-313

[26] Lucendo AJ, Navarro M, Comas C, Pascual JM, Burgos E, Santamaría L, et al. Immunophenotypic characterization and quantification of the epithelial inflammatory infiltrate in eosinophilic esophagitis through stereology: An analysis of the cellular mechanisms of the disease and the immunologic capacity of the esophagus. The American Journal of Surgical Pathology [Internet]. 2007;**31**(4):598-606. Available from: https://pubmed.ncbi.nlm.nih.gov/17414108/ [Accessed: February 12, 2024]

[27] Rusin S, Covey S, Perjar I, Hollyfield J, Speck O, Woodward K, et al. Determination of esophageal eosinophil counts and other histologic features of eosinophilic esophagitis by pathology trainees is highly accurate. Human Pathology. 2017;**62**:50-55

[28] Straumann A, Spichtin HP, Bucher KA, Heer P, Simon HU. Eosinophilic esophagitis: Red on microscopy, white on endoscopy. Digestion [Internet]. 2004;**70**(2):109-116. Available from: https://pubmed.ncbi.nlm.nih.gov/15383737/ [Accessed: February 12, 2024]

[29] Simon D, Radonjic-Hösli S, Straumann A, Yousefi S, Simon HU. Active eosinophilic esophagitis is characterized by epithelial barrier defects and eosinophil extracellular trap formation. Allergy. 2015;**70**(4):443-452

[30] Nguyen N, Fernando SD, Biette KA, Hammer JA, Capocelli KE, Kitzenberg DA, et al. TGF-β1 alters esophageal epithelial barrier function by attenuation of claudin-7 in eosinophilic esophagitis. Mucosal Immunology. 2018;**11**(2):415-426

[31] Katzka DA, Tadi R, Smyrk TC, Katarya E, Sharma A, Geno DM, et al. Effects of topical steroids on tight junction proteins and spongiosis in esophageal epithelia of patients with eosinophilic esophagitis. Clinical Gastroenterology and Hepatology. 2014;**12**(11):1824-9.e1

[32] Rochman M, Travers J, Abonia JP, Caldwell JM, Rothenberg ME. Synaptopodin is upregulated by IL-13 in eosinophilic esophagitis and regulates esophageal epithelial cell motility and barrier integrity. JCI Insight. 2017;**2**(20):e96789

[33] Azouz NP, Ynga-Durand MA, Caldwell JM, Jain A, Rochman M, Fischesser DM, et al. The antiprotease SPINK7 serves as an inhibitory checkpoint for esophageal epithelial inflammatory responses. Science Translational Medicine. 2018;**10**(444):eaap9736

[34] Arias Á, Vicario M, Bernardo D, Olalla JM, Fortea M, Montalban-Arques A, et al. Toll-like receptors-mediated pathways activate inflammatory responses in the esophageal mucosa of adult eosinophilic esophagitis. Clinical and Translational Gastroenterology. 2018;**9**(4):147

[35] Arias Á, Lucendo AJ. Molecular basis and cellular mechanisms of eosinophilic esophagitis for the clinical practice. Expert Review of Gastroenterology & Hepatology. 2019;**13**(2):99-117

[36] Simon D, Marti H, Heer P, Simon HU, Braathen LR, Straumann A. Eosinophilic

esophagitis is frequently associated with IgE-mediated allergic airway diseases. Journal of Allergy and Clinical Immunology [Internet]. 2005;**115**(5):1090-1092. Available from: https://pubmed.ncbi.nlm.nih.gov/15867873/ [Accessed: February 13, 2024]

[37] Pelz BJ, Wechsler JB, Amsden K, Johnson K, Singh AM, Wershil BK, et al. IgE-associated food allergy alters the presentation of paediatric eosinophilic esophagitis. Clinical and Experimental Allergy. 2016;**46**(11):1431-1440

[38] Okada H, Kuhn C, Feillet H, Bach JF. The "hygiene hypothesis" for autoimmune and allergic diseases: An update. Clinical & Experimental Immunology [Internet]. 2010;**160**(1):1-9. Available from: https://pubmed.ncbi.nlm.nih.gov/20415844/ [Accessed: February 13, 2024]

[39] Rajavelu P, Rayapudi M, Moffitt M, Mishra A, Mishra A. Significance of Para-esophageal lymph nodes in food or aeroallergen-induced iNKT cell-mediated experimental eosinophilic esophagitis. American Journal of Physiology. Gastrointestinal and Liver Physiology. 2012;**302**(7):G645-G654

[40] Rayapudi M, Rajavelu P, Zhu X, Kaul A, Niranjan R, Dynda S, et al. Invariant natural killer T-cell neutralization is a possible novel therapy for human eosinophilic esophagitis. Clinical & Experimental Immunology. 2014;**3**(1):e9

[41] Jyonouchi S, Smith CL, Saretta F, Abraham V, Ruymann KR, Modayur-Chandramouleeswaran P, et al. Invariant natural killer T cells in children with eosinophilic esophagitis. Clinical and Experimental Allergy. 2014;**44**(1):58-68

[42] Kirsch R, Bokhary R, Marcon MA, Cutz E. Activated mucosal mast cells differentiate eosinophilic (allergic) esophagitis from gastroesophageal reflux disease. Journal of Pediatric Gastroenterology and Nutrition. 2007;**44**(1):20-26

[43] Mueller S, Neureiter D, Aigner T, Stolte M. Comparison of histological parameters for the diagnosis of eosinophilic oesophagitis versus gastro-oesophageal reflux disease on oesophageal biopsy material. Histopathology. 2008;**53**(6):676-684

[44] Rothenberg ME, Spergel JM, Sherrill JD, Annaiah K, Martin LJ, Cianferoni A, et al. Common variants at 5q22 associate with pediatric eosinophilic esophagitis. Nature Genetics. 2010;**42**(4):289-291

[45] Allen-Brady K, Firszt R, Fang JC, Wong J, Smith KR, Peterson KA. Population-based familial aggregation of eosinophilic esophagitis suggests a genetic contribution. The Journal of Allergy and Clinical Immunology. 2017;**140**(4):1138-1143

[46] Yang ZC, Yi MJ, Ran N, Wang C, Fu P, Feng XY, et al. Transforming growth factor-β1 induces bronchial epithelial cells to mesenchymal transition by activating the snail pathway and promotes airway remodeling in asthma. Molecular Medicine Reports [Internet]. 2013;**8**(6):1663-1668. Available from: https://pubmed.ncbi.nlm.nih.gov/24126595/ [Accessed: February 13, 2024]

[47] Mukkada VA, Haas A, Maune NC, Capocelli KE, Henry M, Gilman N, et al. Feeding dysfunction in children with eosinophilic gastrointestinal diseases. Pediatrics [Internet]. 2010;**126**(3):e672-e677. Available from: https://pubmed.ncbi.nlm.nih.gov/20696733/ [Accessed: February 2, 2024]

[48] Desai TK, Stecevic V, Chang CH, Goldstein NS, Badizadegan K, Furuta GT. Association of eosinophilic inflammation with esophageal food impaction in adults. Gastrointestinal Endoscopy. 2005;**61**(7):795-801

[49] Kapel RC, Miller JK, Torres C, Aksoy S, Lash R, Katzka DA. Eosinophilic esophagitis: A prevalent disease in the United States that affects all age groups. Gastroenterology. 2008;**134**(5):1316-1321

[50] Dhar A, Haboubi HN, Attwood SE, Auth MKH, Dunn JM, Sweis R, et al. British Society of Gastroenterology (BSG) and British Society of Paediatric Gastroenterology, Hepatology and nutrition (BSPGHAN) joint consensus guidelines on the diagnosis and management of eosinophilic oesophagitis in children and adults. Gut. 2022;**71**(8):1459-1487

[51] Schoepfer AM, Safroneeva E, Bussmann C, Kuchen T, Portmann S, Simon HU, et al. Delay in diagnosis of eosinophilic esophagitis increases risk for stricture formation in a time-dependent manner. Gastroenterology. 2013;**145**(6):1230-1232

[52] Dellon ES, Kim HP, Sperry SLW, Rybnicek DA, Woosley JT, Shaheen NJ. A phenotypic analysis shows that eosinophilic esophagitis is a progressive fibrostenotic disease. Gastrointestinal Endoscopy. 2014;**79**(4):577-85.e4

[53] Lipka S, Kumar A, Richter JE. Impact of diagnostic delay and other risk factors on eosinophilic esophagitis phenotype and esophageal diameter. Journal of Clinical Gastroenterology. 2016;**50**(2):134-140

[54] Kim HP, Vance RB, Shaheen NJ, Dellon ES. The prevalence and diagnostic utility of endoscopic features of eosinophilic esophagitis: A meta-analysis. Clinical Gastroenterology and Hepatology. 2012;**10**(9):988-96.e5

[55] Hirano I, Moy N, Heckman MG, Thomas CS, Gonsalves N, Achem SR. Endoscopic assessment of the oesophageal features of eosinophilic oesophagitis: Validation of a novel classification and grading system. Gut. 2013;**62**(4):489-495

[56] Collins MH, Martin LJ, Alexander ES, Boyd JT, Sheridan R, He H, et al. Newly developed and validated eosinophilic esophagitis histology scoring system and evidence that it outperforms peak eosinophil count for disease diagnosis and monitoring. Diseases of the Esophagus. 2017;**30**(3):1-8

[57] Nelson MJ, Miller FH, Moy N, Zalewski A, Gonsalves N, Gregory DL, et al. Comparison of endoscopy and radiographic imaging for detection of esophageal inflammation and remodeling in adults with eosinophilic esophagitis. Gastrointestinal Endoscopy. 2018;**87**(4):962-968

[58] Gentile N, Katzka D, Ravi K, Trenkner S, Enders F, Killian J, et al. Oesophageal narrowing is common and frequently under-appreciated at endoscopy in patients with oesophageal eosinophilia. Alimentary Pharmacology & Therapeutics. 2014;**40**(11-12):1333-1340

[59] Molina-Infante J, Lucendo AJ. Combining different therapeutic interventions in eosinophilic esophagitis may lead to unreplicable and misleading results. Diseases of the Esophagus. 2016;**29**:1172

[60] Arias A, González-Cervera J, Tenias JM, Lucendo AJ. Efficacy of dietary interventions for inducing histologic remission in patients with eosinophilic esophagitis:

A systematic review and meta-analysis. Gastroenterology. 2014;**146**(7):1639-1648

[61] Lucendo AJ. Meta-analysis-based guidance for dietary Management in Eosinophilic Esophagitis. Current Gastroenterology Reports. 2015;**17**(10):464

[62] Gutiérrez-Junquera C, Fernández-Fernández S, Cilleruelo ML, Rayo A, Echeverría L, Quevedo S, et al. High prevalence of response to proton-pump inhibitor treatment in children with esophageal eosinophilia. Journal of Pediatric Gastroenterology and Nutrition. 2016;**62**(5):704-710

[63] von Arnim U, Biedermann L, Aceves SS, Bonis PA, Collins MH, Dellon ES, et al. Monitoring patients with eosinophilic esophagitis in routine clinical practice - international expert recommendations. Clinical Gastroenterology and Hepatology. 2023;**21**(10):2526-2533

[64] Alexander JA. Topical steroid therapy for eosinophilic esophagitis. Journal of Gastroenterology and Hepatology. 2014;**10**(5):327-329

[65] Dellon ES, Spergel JM. Biologics in eosinophilic gastrointestinal diseases. Annals of Allergy, Asthma & Immunology. 2023;**130**(1):21-27

[66] Dellon ES, Rothenberg ME, Collins MH, Hirano I, Chehade M, Bredenoord AJ, et al. Dupilumab in adults and adolescents with eosinophilic esophagitis. The New England Journal of Medicine. 2022;**387**(25):2317-2330

[67] Warners MJ, Oude Nijhuis RAB, de Wijkerslooth LRH, Smout AJPM, Bredenoord AJ. The natural course of eosinophilic esophagitis and long-term consequences of undiagnosed disease in a large cohort. The American Journal of Gastroenterology. 2018;**113**(6):836-844

[68] Lin Z, Kahrilas PJ, Xiao Y, Nicodème F, Gonsalves N, Hirano I, et al. Functional luminal imaging probe topography: An improved method for characterizing esophageal distensibility in eosinophilic esophagitis. Therapeutic Advances in Gastroenterology. 2013;**6**(2):97-107

[69] Desprez C, Roman S, Leroi AM, Gourcerol G. The use of impedance planimetry (endoscopic functional lumen imaging probe, EndoFLIP(®)) in the gastrointestinal tract: A systematic review. Neurogastroenterology and Motility. 2020;**32**(9):e13980

[70] Eluri S, Tappata M, Huang KZ, Koutlas NT, Robey BS, Fan C, et al. Distal esophagus is the most commonly involved site for strictures in patients with eosinophilic esophagitis. Diseases of the Esophagus. 2020;**33**(2):doz088

Chapter 2

Pulmonary Eosinophilias

Natavan A. Farajova, Irada M. Akhundova, Gulzar R. Aliyeva, Rafiq I. Bayramov, Gulustan H. Babayeva, Sadagat S. Sultanova, Natavan R. Ismailova, Jeyhun M. Ismayilzada, Nargiz N. Huseynova, Fidan N. Gasimova, Zulfu Sh. Gadimova and Konul M. Kerimova

Abstract

Eosinophilia is an increase in the number of eosinophils in the peripheral blood. Among eosinophilias, pulmonary eosinophilias are distinguished, which are manifested by radiological changes and an increased content of eosinophils in the lungs. The basis of pathological changes in pulmonary eosinophilia is the activation of eosinophils. They cause bronchospasm, bronchial hyperreactivity, increased vascular permeability and increased fibrosis processes. In the absence of bronchial hyperreactivity, eosinophils limit the development of allergic reactions, and block and eliminate inflammatory mediators (protective effect). With pathology, such protection is disrupted, and the pool of eosinophils increases and eosinophilia of an inflammatory-destructive nature appears with destruction of the interstitium (cytotoxic effect). The etiology of many pulmonary eosinophilias is unknown; there is a possibility that their occurrence may be influenced by certain medications, parasitic infestations and helminth infections. With many pulmonary eosinophilias, lesions also occur in the skin, bones, blood vessels, hepatobiliary and nervous systems. In the treatment of pulmonary eosinophilia, corticosteroids, interferons, monoclonal antibodies and extracorporeal hemocorrection are used. Symptomatic therapy is prescribed to eliminate the clinical symptoms of the disease and improve the quality of life.

Keywords: pulmonary eosinophilia, inflammatory mediators, eosinophilic pneumonia, eosinophilic infiltration, steroid therapy

1. Introduction

Pulmonary eosinophilia (PE) is a large heterogeneous group of pathological conditions, manifested radiographically by the presence of opacities in the lungs and an increase in the content of eosinophils in the lung tissue and often in the peripheral blood [1–3]. In some cases, PE can be asymptomatic and spontaneously undergo complete reversal, but some forms of PE pose a serious threat to the health and life of patients and require urgent treatment [4, 5].

2. Functions of eosinophils in the human organism

Eosinophils are blood cells with a large arsenal of protective functions. They originate from a common myelopoiesis precursor cell, and their maturation and differentiation are under the control of the thymus [5, 6].

Eosinophil maturation begins in the bone marrow within 34 hours. Then mature eosinophils enter the blood and circulate in it for about 2–4 hours. Then they accumulate in the integumentary tissues of various systems—the submucosal layer of the bronchi, gastrointestinal tract, and urinary system—where their content is 100 times higher in the blood. From these tissues, they are then returned to the bloodstream. In a healthy person, 50–250 eosinophils circulate in 1 microliter of blood. In pathological conditions, namely eosinophilia, the rate of appearance of eosinophils in the peripheral blood accelerates by two times [2, 5].

Migration and activation of eosinophils occurs under the influence of various chemotactic factors, including interleukin-5, immune complexes, and activated components of the complement system. Activation of eosinophils ends with their degranulation with the release into the blood of a significant amount of biologically active substances—mediators of allergic inflammation—with a wide spectrum of action. These substances are represented by the main macroprotein with significant toxic and destructive effects, free oxygen radicals—products of the inflammatory process, growth factors, platelet-activating factor, eicosanoids, pro-inflammatory cytokines, and others. Activated eosinophils have a wide range of biological effects (bronchospasm, bronchial hyperreactivity, increased vascular permeability, and increased fibrosis processes in tissues) [2, 4]. If there is no bronchial hyperreactivity, eosinophils limit the development of allergic processes by blocking and eliminating inflammatory mediators. This is reflected in their protective effect, which manifests itself in most allergic diseases. At the same time, during pathological processes, such a protective function is distorted, and the pool of eosinophils increases significantly, contributing to the appearance of eosinophilia.

Thus, in various situations, activation of eosinophils can be both physiological, protective (allergic reactions and helminth infestations) and pathological, and inflammatory and destructive in nature (pulmonary eosinophilia and granulomatous processes) [1, 7]. In these cases, eosinophils act as effector cells that cause the destruction of interstitial tissue. This is confirmed by numerous studies proving the cytotoxic effect of these cells. It is due to this effect that destructive changes occur in the lung parenchyma.

There are two known ways of lung damage in PE: the first way is the destruction of type I and III collagen due to collagenesis, the second way is damage to parenchyma cells due to granular proteins and free oxygen radicals.

3. Classification of PE

There is no generally accepted classification of PE. All PE are usually divided according to the etiological factor and clinical manifestations of the disease [6, 8, 9].

Based on clinical manifestations, the following six forms of the disease.

1. Simple eosinophilic pneumonia (SEP);

2. Acute eosinophilic pneumonia (AEP);

3. Chronic eosinophilic pneumonia (CEP);

4. Idiopathic hypereosinophilic syndrome (IHS);

5. Eosinophilic granulomatosis with polyangiitis (EGPA; Churg-Strauss syndrome);

6. Langerhans cell histiocytosis (LCH; Pulmonary granulomatosis, Histiocytosis X)

Based on origin (etiology), there are five forms of the disease:

1. Idiopathic PE

2. Allergic bronchopulmonary mycoses

3. PE for helminthiasis

4. Medicinal PEs

5. Food PE

4. Epidemiology of PE

PE is a rare disease. Parasitic eosinophilic pneumonias are common in regions where certain parasites are endemic.

Acute eosinophilic pneumonia develops at any age, even in previously healthy children, although the disease is most often observed in patients aged 20–40 years. Men are affected approximately twice as often as women. Acute eosinophilic pneumonia is associated with smoking. Chronic eosinophilic pneumonia develops more often in women than in men and is not associated with smoking. The relationship of the disease with radiation therapy for breast cancer is described [6, 8].

5. Eosinophilic pneumonia

Eosinophilic pneumonia (EP) is a disease accompanied by the accumulation of blood eosinophils in the pulmonary alveoli. There are several types of EP observed. The most common clinical manifestations of the disease are cough, fever, shortness of breath, and night sweats [7, 9]. The diagnosis of eosinophilic pneumonia is made on the basis of the clinical picture, objective examination data, blood counts, and radiological symptoms. Most types of eosinophilic pneumonia are recognizable and treatable with corticosteroids, and the prognosis is good [9, 10].

In this section, we will consider only six clinical forms of EP.

5.1 Simple eosinophilic pneumonia

The most common causes of simple eosinophilic pneumonia (SEP) or Loeffler's syndrome are helminths, drugs, and fungal infections. There are Loeffler I (eosinophilic volatile pulmonary infiltrate) and Loeffler II (restrictive cardiomyopathy).

In ICD-10, the disease is designated by code J82. 41.42: Eosinophilic asthma, Loeffler's pneumonia. This syndrome is recorded in all countries, but most often in tropical climates. The frequency is the same among women and men, mainly occurring between the ages of 16 and 40 years [10, 11].

The disease may be asymptomatic and resolve spontaneously. Patients often experience a dry, unproductive cough, wheezing in the chest, mostly in upper parts, and a feeling of mild pain in the trachea, which is associated with irritation of mucosa during the passage of roundworm larvae or other parasites. The sputum is viscous and may have a slight bloody tint. X-ray examination of the lungs reveals bilateral round or oval infiltrates from several millimeters to several centimeters.

They are accompanied by an increase in the content of EP in peripheral blood by up to 10%. An increased content of EP and their degradation products—Charcot-Leyden crystals—is found in sputum. The level of IgE in the blood is usually elevated (more than 1000 IU/ml). Infiltrates in the lungs persist for several weeks, can migrate across the pulmonary fields, and resolve on their own without residual changes [12].

5.2 Acute eosinophilic pneumonia

Acute eosinophilic pneumonia (AEP) is one of the forms of pulmonary eosinophilia of unknown etiology (sometimes cases of the disease after taking aminopenicillins, tranquilizers, and other drugs) with acute manifestations of intoxication and respiratory symptoms. In severe cases, acute respiratory failure is possible [12, 13]. AEP is characterized by fever, attacks of shortness of breath, muscle, and pleural pain. Shortness of breath during the disease is associated with eosinophilic infiltration of the walls of the bronchi, the accumulation of eosinophils in the alveoli. When auscultating the lungs during the inhalation phase, moist fine rales are mainly heard. On a radiograph (more clearly on CT), merging areas of alveolar infiltration (ground glass symptom) with compaction of the interlobar septa and pleural effusion are detected (pleural effusion).

Laboratory test results reveal eosinophilia in the blood and lavage fluid in 25% of cases.

5.3 Chronic eosinophilic pneumonia

A disease with a chronic course, which is characterized by infiltration of the alveolar walls and pulmonary interstitium by eosinophils, as well as their accumulation in the lumen of the alveoli, the formation of microabscesses and bronchiolitis [13, 14]. The disease often appears after 50 years of age, develops gradually, the first symptoms, often appearing 3–5 months after the onset of the disease, are fever, general weakness, weight loss due to lack of appetite, shortness of breath and cough.

The etiology of chronic eosinophilic pneumonia (CEP) has not been studied.

A study of external respiration function reveals a mixed type of ventilation disorder. X-ray examination reveals bilateral infiltrates in the lateral and cortical areas of the lungs, more in the upper and middle sections [14–16]. Over time, the shadows become more pronounced, sometimes disappear and reappear, i.e. are of a volatile nature.

These changes are more clearly noted on computed tomography (CT).

When examining bronchoalveolar lavage fluid, eosinophilia is detected in more than 40% of cases, confirming the diagnosis of CEP [15, 16]. Histological examination of biopsy material against the background of slight fibrosis reveals eosinophils and histiocytes, as well as multinucleated giant cells.

5.4 Idiopathic hypereosinophilic syndrome

Idiopathic hypereosinophilic syndrome (IHES) is characterized by prolonged, more than 6 months, eosinophilia and eosinophilic infiltration of organs and tissues, which contributes to the characteristic multiple organ damage. The diagnosis of the disease is made on the basis of these symptoms, subject to the exclusion of eosinophilia of other etiologies (parasitic infestations, allergic diseases, and other causes of eosinophilia) [17]. The clinical picture of the disease is dominated by general malaise, muscle pain, dry cough, urticaria and/or angioedema (Quincke's edema). In 80% or more cases, the nervous, cardiovascular, and digestive systems are involved in the process, vision deteriorates, and the hepatobiliary system is affected. Very high leukocytosis is noted. Heart damage often causes disability and indicates an unfavorable prognosis (death may occur) [17, 18]. The severity of the condition is also due to damage to the membranes of the heart in the form of eosinophilic endomyocarditis. In the final stage of the disease, aseptic microabscesses and necrosis form. As a result of the development of necrotic processes and thromboembolic complications, restrictive cardiomyopathy can form [19].

When thromboembolic complications occur in the vessels of the brain, symptoms of encephalitis and/or peripheral neuropathy appear. Manifestations of stroke or transient ischemic disorders are also possible. Embolic complications are often recurrent even during anticoagulant therapy. Encephalopathy in the clinic is manifested by a decrease in intelligence, memory, increased muscle tone, and gait disturbance (ataxia). The appearance of impaired sensation in the limbs and muscle atrophy in patients are symptoms of peripheral neuropathy [18, 19].

A serious problem with IHES is the skin manifestations of the disease in the form of angioedema, erythematous and urticarial rashes, and severe skin itching. The reason for such changes is associated with perivascular eosinophilic infiltration of the skin. From the respiratory system, shortness of breath and an unproductive cough are often noted. X-ray examination often reveals infiltrates resulting from migration of EF into the lung parenchyma. In the later stages of the disease, fibrosis of the lung tissue or infarction pneumonia may develop.

5.5 Eosinophilic granulomatosis with polyangiitis

Eosinophilic granulomatosis with polyangiitis (EGPA) or Churg-Strauss syndrome (CSS) belongs to the group of eosinophilic granulomatosis with damage to the respiratory tract (eosinophilic bronchial asthma) and necrotizing vasculitis with damage to medium and small vessels [20]. The disease was first noted at the beginning of the last century. Later, in 1951, two pathologists Jacob Churg and Lotte Strauss described the clinicopathological signs of the disease on 13 patients, which was named in their honor—Churg-Strauss syndrome (CSS) [20]. The main manifestations in the examined patients were symptoms of severe bronchial asthma, fever, high eosinophilia, polyneuropathy, and heart and kidney failure. Many patients had pulmonary infiltrates, arterial hypertension, sinusitis, abdominal pain, and skin lesions in the form of purpura and subcutaneous nodes. The authors described the morphological triad of the syndrome as—necrotizing vasculitis, eosinophilic tissue infiltration and extravascular granulomas. Subsequently, it was found that EGPA also applies to necrotizing vasculitis associated with antineutrophil cytoplasmic antibodies (ANCA).

According to an international consensus decision in 1992, Charge-Strauss syndrome was classified as a systemic vasculitis affecting small vessels. In 2012, the nomenclature of systemic vasculitides was revised and Charge-Strauss syndrome was replaced by the term "eosinophilic granulomatosis with polyangiitis" and began to refer to 21 groups of ANCA-associated vasculitis. EGPA is characterized by necrotizing granulomatous inflammation, predominantly affecting the respiratory tract, and necrotizing vasculitis, mainly of small and medium vessels, associated with asthma and eosinophilia. Only the upper or lower respiratory tract can be involved in the pathological process. ANCA is found in only 40% of patients with EGPA. Most often, ANCA is determined with glomerulonephritis, and most patients have a history of necrotizing glomerulonephritis [21, 22].

There are two hypotheses regarding the role of ANCA in the development of vasculitis.

According to the first hypothesis, antigens are released from granules of neutrophils or from lysosomes of monocytes, which are perceived by the body's immune system as foreign. These antigens bind to the vascular wall and form antigen-antibody immune complexes. This complex triggers the complement system—protective proteins that participate in the body's immune response. If the immune complex enters a cell, complement proteins destroy its membrane. When there are too many antibody-antigen complexes in the body, they accumulate in small vessels (for example, in the vessels of the skin) and cause local inflammation.

According to the second hypothesis, ANCA interact with neutrophils, which begin to damage vascular endothelial cells. ANCA-activated neutrophils additionally produce proinflammatory cytokines, which initiate an inflammatory response, which causes vascular damage [23]. In individuals with EGPA, pANCA titers have been shown to correlate with disease severity; a decrease in the titers of these antibodies reflected the effectiveness of the immunosuppressive therapy and, conversely, an increase in pANCA titers was considered as a sign of exacerbation of the disease [24, 25]. It has been shown that in individuals with EGPA, ANCA titers correlate with severity of the disease; the decrease in titers of these antibodies reflected the effectiveness ongoing immunosuppressive therapy and, conversely, an increase in pANCA titers was considered as a sign of exacerbation of the disease.

Depending on the presence of ANCA, two types of vasculitis are distinguished: ANCA-positive and ANCA-negative vasculitis.

ANCA-positive vasculitis is characterized by the development of glomerulonephritis, multiple mononeuritis (simultaneous or sequential damage to more than one group of nerves), and frequent exacerbations [26–28].

ANCA-negative vasculitis is characterized by a poorer prognosis associated with a high incidence of cardiomyopathy [29, 30].

EGPA is classified as a rare disease. According to epidemiological studies, the annual incidence per one million population is 0.5–6.8 cases [21, 31–33]. The disease is more common in northern latitudes at any age without gender differences [21, 34]. According to some authors, men get sick 1.3 times more often [35]. There are known cases of the disease in children and adolescents. SES also occurs in old age [36].

The etiology of development and pathogenesis of EGPA have not been fully studied, since the diagnosis of this disease, according to the criteria of the American College of Rheumatology, is carried out not in the early stages of its development, but much later, when the etiological and late trigger factors overlap each other, which makes correct diagnosis difficult, determining the reasons for its development [37]. The most likely etiological factors for this syndrome are genetic causes.

First of all, this is a polymorphism of genes encoding the synthesis of pro- and anti-inflammatory cytokines, antinuclear, and antineutrophil cytoplasmic antibodies

(ANCA) and their physiological inhibitors [38, 39]. A connection between Churg-Strauss syndrome and certain antigens of the HLA-DR3 and HLA-DQ systems has been revealed [39].

EGPA is an idiopathic autoimmune process, but there are certain factors associated with the occurrence of this syndrome. Among them, we can note a drug based on monoclonal antibodies in the treatment of severe bronchial asthma (omalizumab), glucocorticosteroids, leukotriene receptor antagonists, and macrolides [40, 41]. Although a hereditary predisposition to SSS has not been noted, the results of genetic studies have shown the involvement of a number of predisposing hereditary factors, in particular, the interleukin IL10 haplotype-IL10.2, which is associated with increased expression of IL10 [42]; allelic variants of HLA-DRB1*04 and HLA-DRB1*07 and the HLA-DRB4 gene, which are more often detected in patients with SHS than in healthy individuals; and, possibly, the CD226 Gly307Ser polymorphism [43].

In the clinic, the disease is divided into three phases [44].

Phase 1—a combination of two respiratory allergies: bronchial asthma and allergic rhinitis, and recurrent sinusitis and polliposis [45]. Eosinophilic infiltrates in organs (in the lungs—eosinophilic pneumonia, reminiscent of chronic eosinophilic pneumonia).

Phase 2—the appearance of respiratory and extra-respiratory eosinophilic infiltrates.

Phase 3—the predominance of general symptoms in the clinical picture—intoxication, weight loss, myalgia, arthralgia, and general weakness.

The third phase of the disease usually occurs no earlier than 3 years later, and sometimes the manifestation of this phase can last more than one decade. This phase of the disease is characterized by systemic small vessel vasculitides combined with granulomatous infiltration.

The classic course of EGPA begins with damage to the upper respiratory tract (allergic rhinitis, often accompanied by polypous growths of the nasal mucosa). Simultaneously or later, bronchial asthma develops with frequent and severe attacks of broncho-obstructive syndrome [45]. This condition can last for years. Subsequently, eosinophilic infiltrates appear in the lungs and other organs. The final stage in the clinical picture of the syndrome is general symptoms—weakness, intoxication, weight loss, myalgia, and arthralgia.

From the peripheral nerves, multiple mononeuritis or asymmetric polyneuropathy are detected. The development of eosinophilic myocarditis, coronary arteritis, and pericarditis indicate an unfavorable prognosis of the disease. This prognosis is facilitated by the fact that these changes are detected already at the stage of heart failure (left ventricular failure and dilated cardiomyopathy) [24].

Common symptoms are fever, weight loss, arthralgia and myalgia, and weakness.

Thus, during the course of the disease, the following three stages can be roughly distinguished: the development of bronchial asthma and rhinitis, eosinophilic infiltrates in organs and, finally, vasculitis with extrapulmonary manifestations. In 3/4 of patients, allergic rhinitis occurs, combined with recurrent sinusitis and polyposis [45].

In 1/3 of patients, changes in the gastrointestinal tract are detected: gastric and duodenal ulcers, ulcerative colitis, cholecystitis, which are manifested by abdominal pain, diarrhea and may be complicated by bleeding or perforation [2, 46].

In 1/4, moderately severe kidney pathology is determined [46]. Patients with EGPA are characterized by anemia and an increase in ESR. Blood eosinophilia usually reaches 5–20 × 109/L, but can be higher [5]. High levels of eosinophilic neurotoxin in urine are also a marker of EGPA activity [30].

Diagnosis of EGPA is based on the results of clinical, laboratory, and instrumental studies. Due to the paucity of clinical data, the main attention is paid to changes obtained as a result of visualization of the upper respiratory tract (rhinoscopy, laryngoscopy, etc.), as well as methods of radiological diagnosis of the bronchopulmonary system—radiography and computed tomography of the lungs (CT). But it should be noted that X-ray examination is not always informative.

According to CT data, in 70% of cases at different stages of the disease, recurrent pulmonary eosinophilic infiltrates of various shapes and localization are detected. Typically, these infiltrates respond easily to steroid therapy (disappear quickly).

Sometimes an X-ray examination can reveal a combination of pulmonary parenchymal changes with pleural exudate and a change in the size of the heart.

To diagnose SSS, six criteria of the American Rheumatological Association are used:

1. attacks of asthma;
2. eosinophilia more than 10% of the total number of leukocytes;
3. mono- or polyneuropathy;
4. volatile infiltrates in the lungs;
5. sinusitis (clinical and radiological confirmed changes in the paranasal sinuses;
6. accumulation of eosinophils around the vessels determined in biopsy specimens.

The presence of four or more of the six criteria in a patient allows a diagnosis of SSS to be made with a sensitivity of 85% and a specificity of 99%.

5.6 Langerhans cell histiocytosis

LCH (Langerhans cell histiocytosis, eosinophilic granuloma of the lungs, differentiated histiocytosis, histiocytosis X) is a systemic disease characterized by the formation of specific cellular granulomas in various organs and tissues. Pulmonary changes are represented by inflammation of the pulmonary parenchyma with the formation of multiple cysts, manifested by the X-ray picture of a "honeycomb lung" [47]. Frequent localization of the process is the terminal bronchioles and alveoli of the upper and middle sections of the lungs. Sometimes extrapulmonary localization of granulomas is detected in the bones and pituitary gland with the development of diabetes insipidus. Young people aged 20–40 years are most often affected [48, 49]. The main pathogenetic links include the accumulation of Langerhans cells with the restructuring of the bronchial tree and impaired gas exchange [50]. Initially, an X-ray of the lungs reveals small- and medium-sized lesions, thin-walled single cysts located in the upper and middle sections, and the basal sections of the lungs are intact. As it progresses, pneumofibrosis and cystic restructuring increase, spreading to all segments of the lungs [51].

There is no information about the true prevalence of the disease; all that is known is that, thanks to the introduction of open lung biopsy, cases of diagnosing the disease have become more frequent.

The annual incidence of LCH is reported to be 4.6 cases per 1 million children under 15 years of age, with a male to female ratio of 1.2:1 [52].

The estimated incidence in adults is 1–2 cases per million, although LCH is likely underdiagnosed in this population [53]. According to other data, the incidence of LCH is 3–10 cases per 1 million children per year, with its peak occurring between birth and 4 years of age [54]. Boys get sick two times more often [55].

The etiology of LCH is unknown and much controversial. There are assumptions about both the immunological (impaired immune regulation) and the tumor and viral (herpes virus) nature of the disease. It is believed that the herpes virus causes autoaggression of the immune system, in response to which a somatic mutation of the V600E gene encoding the intracellular signaling protein BRAF occurs [56]. In the occurrence of the disease, a number of risk factors are noted, among which a special place is given to tobacco smoking. It has been proven that more than 90% of patients with histiocytosis are smokers [57, 58]. Other risk factors include living in environmentally unfavorable areas, poor nutrition, weak immunity, rheumatism, pulmonary diseases, and chronic inflammatory processes.

The main mechanism of LCH pathogenesis is the accumulation of histiocytes in tissues (dendritic cells-Langerhans cells). Dendritic cells are synthesized in the bone marrow and then migrate to different areas—pulmonary parenchyma, reticuloendothelial system, and dermis [59]. These cells absorb antigens entering the body from the environment and participate in the formation of the immune response. Lymphocytes, as a result of contact with histiocytes, release inflammatory cytokines and substances that activate histiocytes. With pathology (namely with histioitosis X), the process of apoptosis in dendritic cells is disrupted. This process, together with the growth factor secreted by lymphocytes, promotes their intensive proliferation and fusion with eosinophils. Pathological LCH cells actively interact with T-lymphocytes, which leads to the synthesis of a wide range of cytokines and chemokines that contribute to the formation of an inflammatory microenvironment (eosinophils, macrophages, and giant multinucleated osteoclast-like cells) in the lesion [60, 61].

The process ends with the formation of giant cell granulomas. As a result, normal organ tissue is gradually replaced by granulomas with a large number of T-lymphocytes (presumably the presence of a specific antigen).

5.7 Classification of LCH

Langerhans cell histiocytosis is classified according to the location of the lesion and the clinical form of the disease.

By localization of lesions:

- monosystemic form with single or multiple lesions of one anatomical area;
- multisystem form with or without signs of organ dysfunction.

According to clinical the form:

- disseminated form (primary acute, Abt-Letterer-Siwe disease), more often observed in children under 2 years of age, reminiscent of the course of a severe systemic infection, with rapid generalization of the process, progression of respiratory failure and high mortality;
- primary chronic form (Hand-Schüller-Christian disease), a more favorable course, gradual damage to various organs, clinically manifested by Christian's

triad: diabetes insipidus, unilateral exophthalmos, and destruction of the flat bones of the skull, more often observed in children and adolescents;

- eosinophilic granuloma (Taratynov's disease). This is a relatively benign form of the disease with granulomas predominantly localized in the bones and lungs. In most cases, it develops in adults [62].

- The morphological structure of the process is represented by a granuloma, in the center of which there are Langerhans cells, surrounded by layers of eosinophils and lymphocytes. These cells are of monocyte-macrophage origin and are distinguished by a large nucleus and light gray cytoplasm containing granules. Langerhans cells are also found in healthy individuals in the skin, lungs, and pleura. The pathological growth of these cells is observed under the influence of tobacco smoke (in smokers), which increases the concentration of the neuropeptide bombesin, which is produced by neuroendocrine cells.

The clinical picture of LCH is characterized by a gradual onset with poorly expressed symptoms, so a clear identification of the onset of the disease is difficult. The disease in 1/4 of patients occurs completely without any symptoms or changes, primarily without radiological manifestations in the lungs. In 50% of cases in the LCH clinic, a nonproductive cough and decreased tolerance to physical activity appear; in 1/3 of cases, the cough is accompanied by general weakness, fever (low-grade and rarely febrile), and decreased appetite and weight. In some cases, the first manifestations of the disease may be spontaneous, often recurrent pneumothorax. Over time, as the disease progresses, granulomatous changes in the bones, skin, and pituitary gland join the existing symptoms. In the lungs, X-rays reveal reticular nodular infiltrates, localized mainly in the upper and middle zones of the pulmonary fields [63].

CT better visualizes cysts, honeycomb degeneration of lung tissue and their anatomical location, as well as thickening of interstitial tissue.

The result of pulmonary changes in the form of diffuse fibrosis (X-ray picture of the "honeycomb lung") is respiratory failure, pulmonary hypertension, and the formation of chronic pulmonary heart syndrome. From the digestive and hepatobiliary systems, dyspepsia is possible in the form of nausea, vomiting, intestinal dysfunction (mainly diarrhea), dull pain, or heaviness in the right and left hypochondrium (hepato- and splenomegaly). Skin manifestations of the disease in the area of natural folds, as well as the head and ear canal, are observed in the form of hemorrhages and poorly healing ulcers. Some patients may experience bone pain due to osteolysis, manifested by symptoms of tooth loss, unilateral exophthalmos (lysis of the bones of the lower jaw, orbit), in severe cases—bone marrow failure, manifested by anemia with corresponding symptoms (dizziness, pallor of the skin and mucous membranes, and tachycardia). In the presence of granulomas in the posterior lobe of the pituitary gland, symptoms of diabetes insipidus (polydipsia, polyuria, and dry mouth) appear due to insufficiency of antidiuretic hormone [47, 59].

Among the complications of LCH, it is necessary to note a compression fracture of the spine, pulmonary hypertension, spontaneous pneumothorax (rupture of pulmonary bullae in the cortical zones), cirrhosis of the liver with liver failure. In rare cases, as consequences of diabetes insipidus (hyperosmolar hypohydration)—motor restlessness, muscle cramps, and coma [64].

Diagnosis of LCH is based on objective research data, as well as the results of laboratory, radiological and functional research methods. Pay attention to the presence of signs of respiratory failure (diffuse cyanosis of the skin, tension in the respiratory muscles); data from auscultation of the lungs (hard or weakened hard breathing with bilateral widespread dry rales of various sizes throughout all pulmonary fields); laboratory blood test data (increased erythrocyte sedimentation rate—ESR, eosinophilia, pancytopenia, increased liver enzymes, increased plasma osmolarity, prolongation of prothrombin time, and hypofibrinogenemia in liver failure) [63, 64].

X-ray examination reveals foci of osteolysis and destruction in the tubular bones and bones of the skull. On the X-ray of the lungs, against the background of an intensified pulmonary pattern, bilateral small-focal darkening is detected. A more informative method of radiodiagnosis is computed tomography (CT) and high-resolution CT (HRCT), which allows one to determine fibrosis of the pulmonary parenchyma.

A study of the function of external respiration (spirography and body plethysmography) reveals restrictive disorders of the ventilation function of the lungs with a decrease in their total capacity and elasticity indicators, as well as a decrease in the diffusion capacity of the lungs (DLco), which increases with physical activity.

Histological examination of a biopsy of the skin, lymph nodes, or lungs reveals an excessive number of giant Langerhans cells with eosinophilic cytoplasm, a bean-shaped nucleus, and the absence of nucleoli [65, 66].

In the generalized form of LCH, differential diagnosis is carried out mainly with acute leukemia, hemophagocytic syndrome, hyperparathyroidism, myeloma, osteomyelitis (with bone destruction), as well as skin allergies (eczema, atopic dermatitis, and psoriasis).

Pulmonary manifestations of the disease must be differentiated from tuberculosis and pulmonary sarcoidosis, lymphogranulomatosis, and fibrosing processes of another etiology.

6. Treatment of PE

6.1 Treatment of SEP

Treatment is mainly aimed at eliminating the causative factor: stopping the etiologically significant medication, deworming, and therapy for pulmonary mycosis. Conservative treatment also includes bronchodilators. Usually, due to the spontaneous resolution of pulmonary infiltrates, glucocorticosteroids (GCS) are not prescribed. But sometimes, a short treatment regimen with small doses of corticosteroids is used—20–25 mg/day prednisolone for 1 week, which leads to the rapid and complete disappearance of PEP symptoms. The prognosis of the disease is favorable.

6.2 Treatment of AEP

If a causative factor is detected, treatment is aimed at it and the administration of large doses of corticosteroids—prednisolone 2 mg/kg per day leads to a rapid and complete recovery without relapses. Initial therapy takes 1–2 weeks, then the daily dose is gradually reduced to 15–20 mg, which can be taken intermittently. The average duration of treatment with GCS is 3 months.

Since most patients with AEP are admitted to the hospital with respiratory failure (RF), initial treatment begins with respiratory support, which includes oxygen therapy and mechanical ventilation (ALV). Patients with AEP respond quickly to treatment with corticosteroids, and in most cases, resolution of the main symptoms is achieved within 1–3 days, and can be quickly disconnected from mechanical ventilation and oxygen therapy. In the vast majority of patients, X-ray changes in the lungs normalize within a week, but mild opacities of the lungs and pleurisy persist on high-resolution computed tomography (HRCT) of the chest for 2 weeks.

Patients on invasive respiratory support (IRS) are prescribed methylprednisolone 60–125 mg IV every 6 hours for 3 days until clinical improvement and extubation, followed by a reduction in the dose of oral prednisolone to 40–60 mg and tapering over 6–12 weeks. A 2-week course of treatment with an initial dose of prednisolone 30 mg per day (or methylprednisolone 60 mg intravenously every 6 hours in patients with DN) is sufficient.

However, the classic 6–12-week treatment regimen is mainly used.

The overall prognosis for AEP after treatment is good, with the disappearance of radiological infiltrates and the absence of long-term pulmonary complications. Unlike CEP, with OEP, after discontinuation of the course of steroid therapy, no relapses of the disease are observed.

6.3 Treatment of CEP

Begin treatment with low doses of corticosteroids (prednisolone 20 mg/day daily or every other day). After 6 months from the start of treatment, when steroid therapy is stopped, there is a high probability of relapse of the disease. This condition requires resumption of treatment, which lasts more than 1 year and is quite effective.

For this form of eosinophilic pneumonia, parenteral (intravenous and oral) administration of steroids is also effective. It must be borne in mind that the lack of effect of treatment makes the diagnosis of CEP questionable and requires further diagnostic search.

Another option for steroid therapy for CEP is the prescription of a high initial dose of prednisolone—from 40 to 60 mg, once a day. Often such treatment leads to surprisingly rapid clinical improvement (sometimes within 2 days). Complete resolution of clinical manifestations and radiological changes occurs within 14 days in most patients and within 1 month in all patients. Therefore, assessing the dynamics of these indicators is a reliable and effective way to monitor the effectiveness of therapy. Although CT is more sensitive in detecting radiological changes, its advantages in assessing the dynamics of the process have not been noted. The number of eosinophils in peripheral blood, ESR, and IgE concentrations can also be used to monitor the clinical course of the disease during treatment. However, not all patients experience pathological changes in laboratory test results.

6.4 Treatment of IHES

GCS for this form of pulmonary eosinophilia is prescribed only at the stage of multiorgan damage. At the initial stages of the disease, when high eosinofolia of the blood is detected and there are no signs of damage to the heart, lungs, nervous system, or skin, it is recommended to limit ourselves to monitoring the patient. GCS therapy, in cases of low effectiveness of prednisolone, is supplemented by the administration of cyclosporine and α-interferon.

It is always possible to completely get rid of the disease. But with the help of modern treatment methods, it is possible to reduce the risk of relapses, prevent irreversible damage to internal organs, and prolong the patient's life.

Therapy uses drugs that affect the level of eosinophils—primarily corticosteroids, interferons, and monoclonal antibodies. To eliminate the clinical symptoms of the disease and improve the quality of life, symptomatic therapy is prescribed.

When treating patients with the myeloproliferative variant of IHES, the first-line drug is imatinib, especially when the recombinant protein FIP1L1-PDGFRA is detected. Discontinuation of the drug does not lead to relapse of the disease. In some patients, low dose imatinib is necessary to maintain long-term remission.

GCS are recommended for the lymphocytic variant of IGES (with a response in only half of the patients) and at the stage of multiorgan damage. If left untreated, restrictive heart failure quickly develops. Other treatments include chemotherapy drugs (hydroxyurea, vincristine, and etoposide), cyclosporine A, JAK kinase inhibitors, alemtuzumab, interferon-α, combination of interferon-α with hydroxyurea for the treatment of myeloproliferative variant, mepolizumab, benralizumab, and dexpramipexole.

The prognosis for idiopathic HES has improved markedly. Thus, the 3-year survival rate is 12%, the 5-year survival rate is 80%, and the 10-year survival rate is 70%. This suggests that advances in molecular biology may provide a better prognosis for patients with previously untreatable disease.

6.5 Treatment of EGPA (CSS)

High doses of systemic corticosteroids are used (prednisolone 1 mg/kg per day).

If there is no immediate effect from GCS, cyclophosphamide (2 mg/kg per day) is added for 6 months. When stabilization is achieved, you can switch to a maintenance dose of prednisolone (up to 20 mg/day).

It is advisable to continue immunosuppressive therapy with cyclophosphamide for up to 1 year, and maintenance monotherapy with prednisone for a long time, depending on the dynamics of the process. Combination therapy improves prognosis, provides 5-year survival in 90%, and 10-year survival in 75% of patients.

As initial treatment for patients with EGPA, pulse therapy with methylprednisolone is used, after which systemic corticosteroids—prednisolone, at a daily dose of 1 mg/kg—are continued for several months followed by dose reduction. In half of the patients, such treatment achieves stable remission [15]. An important indicator of achieving remission is maintaining a blood eosinophilia level of 1 × 109/l [6]. In cases of severe EGPA, ineffectiveness of systemic corticosteroids, development of relapses after discontinuation or reduction of the dose of systemic corticosteroids, therapy is supplemented with the prescription of cytostatics (azathioprine or cyclophosphamide). There is experience with the successful use of interferon and a combination of cyclosporine with intravenous immunoglobulin in patients with severe disease [10].

If the disease is resistant to traditional treatment, a significant improvement in the results of treatment of EGPA can be achieved through the use of modern technologies of extracorporeal hemocorrection [18]. The use of extracorporeal hemocorrection technologies in the treatment of EGPA, which makes it possible to selectively remove pathogenicity factors such as circulating immune complexes and autoaggressive antibodies from the body, makes it possible to significantly improve the results of treatment of this disease. In addition, the use of modern technologies of extracorporeal hemocorrection, as a rule, makes it possible to significantly reduce course doses of corticosteroids and cytostatics [7]. The 5-year survival rate for EGPA is 79% [7, 12].

6.6 Treatment of LCH

There are no generally accepted treatments for LCH. Patients often experience spontaneous remissions. It is necessary to quit smoking and avoid passive smoking. It is usually recommended to prescribe GCS, especially to those patients who have spontaneous pneumothorax or have identified reticular nodular infiltrates in the lungs. Lung transplantation is indicated for patients with honeycomb lung degeneration and severe signs of respiratory failure.

Patients must be hospitalized in a hospital. In severe DN, oxygen inhalation or transfer to mechanical ventilation is indicated. If there are signs of bone marrow failure, they resort to transfusion blood agents and the use of granulocyte colony-stimulating factor.

There is no etiotropic therapy for LCH. The most important stage in treatment is quitting smoking. Quitting smoking causes an improvement in the clinical, laboratory, and radiological picture. GCS (prednisolone and methylprednisolone) and chemotherapeutic agents (vinblastine, mercaptopurine, and etoposide) are used as pathogenetic therapy.

For the treatment of diabetes insipidus, hormone replacement therapy with vasopressin analogues (desmopressin) in the form of an intranasal spray or in tablet form is prescribed. For small osteolytic lesions, curettage is performed; for severe bone infiltration, resection or remote gamma therapy is performed. In case of a massive destructive process in the lung tissue, a lung transplant is performed.

Treatment of the single-system cutaneous form of LCH depends on the extent of the lesion. Local treatment is prescribed, consisting of the use of corticosteroids, mechlorethamine, or phototherapy. Since spontaneous remissions occur, individual lesions require only observation.

For patients with LCH with a single bone lesion, often after a biopsy of the lesion, it is sometimes necessary to curettage the lesion and administer a local steroid or use radiation therapy.

Indications for systemic treatment:

- single-system multifocal and multisystem diseases;
- changes in the bones of the skull and spine (increased risk of involvement of the central nervous system);
- involvement of high-risk organs, i.e. bone marrow, spleen, and liver.

Vinblastine (an anticancer drug) is often used for treatment in combination with prednisolone, in some cases with 6-mercaptopurine. The course of treatment usually lasts 12 months.

If the response to this treatment is unsatisfactory and the disease progresses, other cytostatics are used, for example, cytarabine, cladribine, vincristine, methotrexate, or mercaptopurine.

When a mutation is detected, based on the result of a molecular test, targeted treatments are used, significantly improving the prognosis in the most severe cases.

The prognosis for LCH in children and adults may be different. The disease may disappear spontaneously or develop into a disseminated form that is life-threatening.

In the single-system form, the prognosis is good; in the case of the multisystem form, it depends on the affected organs. Involvement of the central nervous system, bone marrow, liver, and spleen significantly worsen the prognosis.

DOI: http://dx.doi.org/10.5772/intechopen.1005831

Author details

Natavan A. Farajova[1*], Irada M. Akhundova[2], Gulzar R. Aliyeva[2], Rafiq I. Bayramov[3], Gulustan H. Babayeva[1], Sadagat S. Sultanova[1], Natavan R. Ismailova[1], Jeyhun M. Ismayilzada[3], Nargiz N. Huseynova[1], Fidan N. Gasimova[1], Zulfu Sh. Gadimova[3] and Konul M. Kerimova[4]

1 Department of Therapy, Azerbaijan State Institute for Advanced Training of Doctors, Ministry of Health Azerbaijan Republic, Baku, Azerbaijan

2 Scientific Research Institute of Lung Diseases, Ministry of Health Azerbaijan Republic, Baku, Azerbaijan

3 Department of Lung Diseases, Azerbaijan Medical University, Ministry of Health Azerbaijan Republic, Baku, Azerbaijan

4 Science, Scientific Research Institute of Lung Diseases, Ministry of Health Azerbaijan Republic, Baku, Azerbaijan

*Address all correspondence to: natavanfa@mail.ru

References

[1] Carbone RG, Puppo F, Mattar E, Roden AC, Hirani N. Acute and chronic eosinophilic pneumonia: An overview. Frontiers in Medicine (Lausanne). 22 Apr 2024;**11**:1355247. DOI: 10.3389/fmed.2024.1355247

[2] Voitsekhovskiy VV, Landyshev YS, Tseluyko SS. Eosinophilia. Amurskiy meditsinskiy zhurnal. 2015;**1**:6-17 (in Russian)

[3] Cottin V. Eosinophilic lung diseases. Immunology and Allergy Clinics of North America. 2023;**43**(2):289-322. DOI: 10.1016/j.iac.2023.01.002

[4] Jackson DJ, Wechsler ME, editors. Eosinophilic Lung Diseases (ERS Monograph). Sheffield: European Respiratory Society; 2022. 257p. DOI: 10.1183/2312508X.10029820

[5] Anaev EK. Eosinophils and eosinophilia. Atmosphere Pulmonology and Allergology. 2002;**3**(6):15-18 (in Russian)

[6] Ilkovich MM, editor. Interstitial and Orphan Lung Diseases. Moskva: GEOTAR-Media; 2016. 560 p. (in Russian)

[7] Bartal C, Sagy I, Barski L. Drug-induced eosinophilic pneumonia: A review of 196 case reports. Medicine (Baltimore). 2018;**97**(4):e9688. DOI: 10.1097/MD.0000000000009688

[8] Kogan EA, Kruglikov GG, Tseluyko SS, Sokolina IA, Paukov VS. Pathology of the Respiratory System. Moscow: LitTerra; 2013 (in Russian)

[9] Chuchalin AG. Pulmonology: National Guidelines. Moscow: GEOTAR-Media; 2009, 960 p. (in Russian)

[10] Chuchalin AG. Hypereosinophilia in respiratory diseases. Terapevticheskii arkhiv. 2003;**75**(3):5-15 (in Russian)

[11] Fernandez Perez ER, Olson AL, Frankel SK. Eosinophilic lung diseases. Medical Clinics of North America. 2011;**95**(6):1163-1187

[12] Chuchalin AG. Hypereosinophilia in respiratory diseases. RMJ. 2002;**23**:1047. (In the CEP section) (in Russian)

[13] De Giacomi F, Dekker PA, Vassallo R, Ryu JH. Acute eosinophilic pneumonia: Relationship of clinical characteristics to underlying cause. RIB Cage. 2017;**152**:379-385. DOI: 10.1016/j.chest.2017.03.001

[14] Carbone RG, Puppo F, Mattar E, Rodin AC, Hirani N. Acute and chronic eosinophilic pneumonia: A review. Frontiers in Medicine. 2024;**11**:1355247. DOI: 10.3389/fmed.2024.1355247

[15] Roden AK, Camus P. Iatrogenic lung lesions. Semiotic Diagnosis. 2018;**35**:260-271. DOI: 10.1053/j.semdp.2018.03.002

[16] Mochimaru H, Kawamoto M, Fukuda Y, Kudoh S. Clinicopathological differences between acute and 7 chronic eosinophilic pneumonia. Respirology. 2005;**10**:76-85

[17] Ogbogu PU, Bochener BS, Butterfield HJ, et al. Hypereosinophilic syndromes: A multicenter, retrospective analysis of clinical characteristics and response to therapy. The Journal of Allergy and Clinical Immunology. 2009;**124**:1319-1325

[18] Cordier JF et al. Hypereosinophilic obliterative bronchiolitis: A distinct, unrecognised syndrome. The European Respiratory Journal. 2013;**41**(5):1126-1134

[19] Katre RS et al. Cardiopulmonary and gastrointestinal manifestations of eosinophil-associated diseases and idiopathic hypereosinophilic syndromes: Multimodality imaging approach. Radiographics. 2016;**36**(2):433-451

[20] Jennette JC, Falk RJ, Andrassy K, et al. Nomenclature of systemic vasculitides. Proposal of an international consensus conference. Arthritis and Rheumatism. 1994;**37**:187-192

[21] Mahr A, Guillevin L, Poissonnet M, Ayme S. Prevalences of polyarteritis nodosa, microscopic polyangiitis, Wegener's granulomatosis, and Churg-Strauss syndrome in a French urban multiethnic population in 2000: A capture-recapture estimate. Arthritis and Rheumatism. 2004;**51**(1):92-99

[22] Guillevin L, Cohen P, Gayraud M, et al. Churg-Strauss syndrome. Clinical study and long-term follow-up of 96 patients. Medicine (Baltimore). 1999;**78**:26

[23] Harrold LR, Andrade SE, Go AS, et al. Incidence of Churg-Strauss syndrome in asthma drug users: A population-based perspective. The Journal of Rheumatology. 2005;**32**(6):1076-1080

[24] Wiik A. Autoantibodies in vasculitis. Arthritis Research and Therapy. 2003;**5**(3):147-152

[25] Semenkova EN, Moiseev SV, Namestnikova OG. Clinical aspects of hypereosinophilia syndrome. Klinicheskaia Meditsina. 2004;**2**:28-31 (in Russian)

[26] Sinico RA, Di Toma L, Maggiore U, et al. Prevalence and clinical significance of antineutrophil cytoplasmic antibodies in Churg-Strauss syndrome. Arthritis and Rheumatism. 2005;**52**:2926-2935

[27] Nathani N, Little MA, Kunst H, et al. Churg-Strauss syndrome and leukotriene antagonist use: A respiratory perspective. Thorax. 2008;**63**:883

[28] Keogh KA, Specks U. Churg-Strauss syndrome: Clinical presentation, antineutrophil cytoplasmic antibodies, and leukotriene receptor antagonists. The American Journal of Medicine. 2003;**115**:284

[29] Sablé-Fourtassou R, Cohen P, Mahr A, et al. Antineutrophil cytoplasmic antibodies and the Churg-Strauss syndrome. Annals of Internal Medicine. 2005;**143**:632

[30] Ovcharenko SI, Kapustina VA, Morozova NV. Difficulties in diagnosing Churg-Strauss syndrome. Difficult Patient. 2009;**4-5**:35-38. (in Russian)

[31] Moiseev SV, Semenkova EN, Novikov PI. Current nomenclature of systemic vasculitis—Recommendations of the international consensus conference (Chapel Hill, 2012). Clinical Nephrology. 2012;**2**:41-46 (in Russian)

[32] Sinico RA, Bottero P. Churg-Strauss angiitis. Best Practice and Research: Clinical Rheumatology. 2009;**23**:355-366

[33] Pagnoux C, Guillevin L. Churg-Strauss syndrome: Evidence for disease subtypes? Current Opinion in Rheumatology. 2010;**22**:21-28

[34] Kahn JE, Bletry O, Guillevin L. Hypereosinophilic syndromes. Best Practice and Research: Clinical Rheumatology. 2008;**22**:863-882

[35] Chuchalina AG, editor. Pulmonology: National Leadership. Moscow: GEOTAR-Media; 2009. 960 p. (in Russian)

[36] Nasonov EL, Baranov AA, Shilkina NP. Vasculitis and Vasculopathy. Yaroslavl: Upper Volga; 1999. 616 p. (in Russian)

[37] Palange P, Rohde G, editors. ERS Handbook of Respiratory Medicine. 3rd ed. AfkEbooks; 2019. 886 p. DOI: 10.1183/9781849840798. ISBN 9781849840798

[38] Yudin AA, Kurbacheva OM, Poletaeva TA, Azerkovich VN. Differential diagnosis of bronchial asthma and Churg-Strauss syndrome (analysis of clinical observation). Pulmonology. 2010;**1**:115-117 (in Russian)

[39] Avdeev SN, Karchevskaya NA, Zubairova PA. Churg-Strauss syndrome as a cause of refractory bronchial asthma. Pulmonology and Allergology. 2012;**1**:42-44 (in Russian)

[40] Wechsler ME, Wong DA, Miller MK, Lawrence-Miyasaki L. Churg–Strauss syndrome in patients treated with omalizumab. Chest. 2009;**136**:507-518

[41] Hauser T, Mahr A, Metzler C, et-al. The leucotriene recetor antagonist montelukast and the risk of Churg–Strauss syndrome: A case-crossover study. Thorax. 2008;**63**:677-682

[42] Vaglio A, Martorana D, Maggiore U, et al. HLA-DRB4 as a genetic risk factor for Churg-Strauss syndrome. Arthritis and Rheumatism. 2007;**56**:3159-3166

[43] Wieczorek S, Holle JU, Epplen JT. Recent progress in the genetics of Wegener's granulomatosis and Churg-Strauss syndrome. Current Opinion in Rheumatology. 2010;**22**(1):8-14

[44] Lanham JG, Elkon KB, Pusey CD, Hughes GR. Systemic vasculitis with asthma and eosinophilia: A clinical approach to the Churg–Strauss syndrome. Medicine (Baltimore). 1984;**63**:65-81

[45] Chervyakova GA, Kozlova NP, Fung ZS. Churg-Strauss syndrome. Lechebnoe delo. 2007;**2**:97-99 (in Russian)

[46] Katzenstein AL. Diagnostic features and differential diagnosis of Churg-Strauss syndrome in the lung: A review. American Journal of Clinical Pathology. 2000;**114**(5):767-772

[47] Latyshev VD, Lukina EA. Langerhans cell Histiocytosis in adults: Treatment opportunities of today. Clinical Oncohematology. 2021;**14**(4):444-454. (In Russ). DOI: 10.21320/2500-2139-2021-14-4-444-454

[48] Allen CE, Ladisch S, McClain KL. How i treat langerhans cell histiocytosis. Blood. 2015;**126**(1):26-35. DOI: 10.1182/blood-2014-12-569301

[49] Shumilin AA, Pavlov AI, Prokhorchik AA, et al. Rare forms of interstitial lung diseases: Clinical case of pulmonary histiocytosis X. Effective Pharmacotherapy. 2023;**19**(20):26-31. DOI: 10.33978/2307-3586-2023-19-20-26-31 (in Russian)

[50] Friedman B, Cronstein B. Methotrexate mechanism in treatment of rheumatoid arthritis. Joint Bone Spine. 2019;**86**(3):301-307. DOI: 10.1016/j.jbspin.2018.07.004

[51] Steen AE, Steen KH, Bauer R, et al. Successful treatment of cutaneous langerhans cell histiocytosis with low-dose methotrexate. The British Journal of Dermatology. 2001;**145**(1):137-140. DOI: 10.1046/j.1365-2133.2001.04298.x

[52] Weitzman R, Sauter N, Eriksen EF, et al. Critical review: Updated recommendations for the prevention, diagnosis, and treatment of osteonecrosis of the jaw in cancer patients—May 2006. Critical Reviews in Oncology/Hematology. 2007;**62**(2):148-152. DOI: 10.1016/j.critrevonc.2006.12.005

[53] Makras P, Tsoli M, Anastasilakis AD, et al. Denosumab for the treatment of adult multisystem langerhans cell

histiocytosis. Metabolism. 2017;**69**:107-111. DOI: 10.1016/j.metabol.2017.01.004

[54] Volkova EN, Bronin GO, Vysotskaya TA, Finogenova NA, Tiganova OA, Nepokul'chitskaya NV, et al. Rezul'taty retrospektivnogo monotsentrovogo issledovaniya gistiotsitoza iz kletok Langergansa u detey. Pediatriya. Zhurn. im. G.N. Speranskogo. 2009;**87**(4):33-40. (in Russian)

[55] Goyal G, Tazi A, Go RS, Rech KL, Picarsic JL, Vassallo R, et al. International expert consensus recommendations for the diagnosis and treatment of Langerhans cell histiocytosis in adults. Blood. 28 Apr 2022;**139**(17):2601-2621. DOI: 10.1182/blood.2021014343

[56] Badalian-Very G, Vergilio J-A, Degar BA, et al. Recurrent BRAF mutations in langerhans cell histiocytosis. Blood. 2010;**116**(11):1919-1923. DOI: 10.1182/blood-2010-04-279083

[57] Colby TV, Lombard C. Histiocytosis X in the lung. Human Pathology. 1983;**14**:847-856

[58] Mogulkoc N, Veral A, Bishop PW, et al. Pulmonary langerhans' cell histiocytosis: Radiologic resolution follow$ ing smoking cessation. Chest. 1999;**115**(5):1452-1455

[59] Collin M, Bigley V, McClain KL, et al. Cell(s) of origin of langerhans cell histiocytosis. Hematology/Oncology Clinics of North America. 2015;**29**(5):825-838. DOI: 10.1016/j.hoc.2015.06.003

[60] Allen CE, Beverley PCL, Collin M, et al. The coming of age of langerhans cell histiocytosis. Nature Immunology. 2020;**21**(1):1-7. DOI: 10.1038/s41590-019-0558-z

[61] Allen CE, Merad M, McClain KL. Langerhans-cell histiocytosis. The New England Journal of Medicine. 2018;**379**(9):856-868. DOI: 10.1056/NEJMra1607548

[62] Burtsev EA, Bronin GO. Langerhans cell histiocytosis in children: Literature review. Voprosy sovremennoi pediatrii — Current Pediatrics. 2023;**22**(1):13-22. (In Russ). DOI: 10.15690/vsp.v22i1.2520

[63] Kornev BM, Kogan EA, Popov EN, et al. Pulmonary histiocytosis X—Modern concepts, diagnosis and treatment tactics. Therapeutic Archive. 2003;**78**(3):68-72 (in Russian)

[64] Potapenko VG, Baykov VV, Zinchenko AV, Potikhonova NA. Langerhans cell histiocytosis in adults: Literature review. Onkogematologiya—Oncohematology. 2022;**17**(4):16-32. (in Russian). DOI: 10.17650/1818-8346-2022-17-4-16-32

[65] Auerswald U, Barth J, Magnussen H. Value of CD-1-positive cells in bronchoalveolar lavage fluid for the diagnosis of pulmonary histiocytosis X. Lung. 1991;**169**(6):305-309. DOI: 10.1007/BF02714167

[66] Girschikofsky M, Arico M, Castillo D, et al. Management of adult patients with langerhans cell histiocytosis: Recommendations from an expert panel on behalf of euro-histio-net. Orphanet Journal of Rare Diseases. 2013;**8**:72. DOI: 10.1186/1750-1172-8-72

Chapter 3

Navigating the Terrain: Type 2 Cytokines and Biologic Intervention in Severe Eosinophilic Asthma

Brian W.P. Seymour, Ashley A. Seymour and Patricia M. Gilford

Abstract

Asthma is a chronic respiratory disease characterized by bronchial hyperreactivity. There are several endotypes of which allergic asthma is the most common. Severe eosinophilic asthma is prevalent in approximately 5% of asthmatics and its phenotype overlaps with allergic asthma and type 2 inflammation. Patients with refractiveness to corticosteroids underline the difficulty in controlling persistent inflammation in severe eosinophilic asthma. The focus of biological therapies is geared towards the understanding of the intricate interplay of the cytokines that drive the eosinophil's ability to induce chronic inflammation with airway obstruction. This chapter takes the reader down a historical journey of initial studies that were performed using mouse helper T cell clones for reconstitution experiments to unravel the mechanism of the role T helper 2 cytokines play in allergic asthma. We then reviewed the classic in vivo experiments that demonstrated how antibodies to IL5 can down regulate eosinophils in the blood and their progenitors in the bone marrow of mice. We also delve into the complex interaction of the alarmins on the cytokines triggers of allergic inflammation with elevated eosinophils. Finally, we review the clinical literature on the beneficial effects of humanized monoclonal antibodies in use for treatment of patients suffering from severe eosinophilic asthma.

Keywords: cytokine, antibody, alarmin, asthma, eosinophil, inflammation

1. Introduction

Asthma is a chronic respiratory disease characterized by bronchial hyperreactivity (narrowing of the airways), wheezing and tightness of the chest [1, 2]. It affects more than 300 million people worldwide with approximately 25 million in the United States [3–6]. It is one of the most chronic diseases in children with the morbidity and mortality rates highest among African American children in the United States [7]. They are at least 10 times more likely to die from asthma than their white counterparts [7–9]. It is a complex and heterogenous disease with varying severity that has a great spectrum of symptoms and wide differences in treatment efficacy [10]. The future in asthma management is to classify its many patterns known as endotypes, that connect recognizable characteristics with immunological mechanisms [5]. These endotypes can range from allergic bronchopulmonary aspergillosis, viral-exacerbated asthma, exercise-induced asthma to allergic and eosinophilic asthma [5, 10, 11].

Allergic asthma is the most common endotype as it affects approximately 66% of patients with asthma and more than half of the patients with severe asthma [12]. It is characterized by elevated levels of serum IgE (>0.35kU/L) with specificity for allergens in sensitized individuals [13]. These allergens are often innocuous and ubiquitous such as the antigens in house dust mites, pollen, dog and or cat dander. Atopic individuals diagnosed with allergic asthma show a positive skin prick test to allergens along with bronchial hyper-responsiveness and elevated levels of blood eosinophils [13].

Eosinophilia of the airways is observed in greater than 50% of all asthmatics. Those patients with sputum eosinophilia ($\geq$3%) and blood eosinophil levels of $\geq$300cells/μl are designated as having severe eosinophilic asthma [13, 14]. High blood eosinophil count is a risk factor for asthma [15, 16]. Individuals exposed to tobacco smoke as well as ex-smokers have significantly higher levels of eosinophils when compared to non-smokers [17]. Indeed, in a murine model of asthma, mice exposed to environmental tobacco smoke had significantly higher levels of blood eosinophils and increases in bronchial hyperreactivity when compared to those exposed to filtered air [18]. Patients with prolonged eosinophilic asthma will have an accumulation of eosinophils not only in the blood and sputum but also in the bronchial tract. These patients will have a basement membrane zone of the airways that is thickened. Here, eosinophils will produce cytokines, chemokines and other mediators of inflammation [19] resulting in airway obstruction and airway remodeling [20]. This remodeling results in subepithelial fibrosis, thickening of the sub-basement membrane, increase airway smooth muscle mass and mucous gland hyperplasia with consequences of asthma exacerbation [19]. The Global Initiative for Asthma (GINA) describes asthma exacerbation as the inability of an asthmatic to respond to inhaled corticosteroids (ICS) due to high levels of inflammation in the airways with consequences of tightness of the chest, wheezing and decrease in lung function [21].

The European Academy of Allergy and Clinical Immunology Biological Guidelines from 2020 states that allergic asthma and eosinophilic asthma are subtypes of a type 2 (T2)—high inflammation [22]. A T2 high phenotype is characteristic of patients with high levels of blood eosinophil and IL5 in bronchial biopsies. A common biomarker for a T2-high inflammation is a fractional exhaled nitric oxide (FeNO) of $\geq$35 ppb [13]. Clinical studies show that many of these patients met the definition of both allergic and eosinophilic asthma demonstrating overlapping characteristics between both groups [13, 23]. Severe eosinophilic asthma patients will express a T2-high asthma phenotype with a biomarker of FeNO of $\geq$35 ppb [13]. These patients also exhibit a T helper (Th)2 cytokine profile (IL4, IL5, IL9, IL13) with IL5 significantly elevated in those with severe asthma [5, 24].

Asthma in many patients is controlled by treatment using standard protocol which includes ICS and beta2 adrenergic bronchodilators [25]. However, 5–10% of patients on corticosteroids do not respond to these medications resulting in persistent inflammation [14]. At center stage of patients with persistent inflammation is the eosinophil and the major cytokine-IL5. IL5 plays the most important role in the growth, differentiation, activation, recruitment and survival of eosinophils [26–28]. Excessive amount of IL5 in the bronchial region is believed to be responsible for the persistent inflammation and the ineffectiveness of corticosteroids in patients with severe eosinophilic asthma [29].

Severe eosinophilic asthma has now become the focus of many new therapies due to the eosinophil's ability to induce chronic airway inflammation, leading to edema, mucus plugging and ultimately airway remodeling and its refractiveness to corticosteroids [30, 31]. The presence of IL5 has been implicated in the prolonged inflammation and remodeling of the airways as shown by several investigators [32–34]. The production of IL5 in this capacity involved a series of complex interactions involving type 2 innate lymphoid cells (ILC2), Th2 cells, the cytokines produced by them and other cells of the immune system. In this chapter, we delve into the early studies (in vitro and in vivo) that paved the way to the understanding of the cytokine functions particularly IL4 and IL5 and the series of intricate interactions that lead to severe eosinophilic asthma. We conclude by discussing the efficacy of biologics in use to treat severe eosinophilia in patients with T2-high asthma.

2. Early in vitro studies helped to unravel the functions of IL4 and IL5

In the early 1980s, investigators from the laboratories of Vitetta used supernatants from a specific T helper cell clone in culture which when added to liposaccharide (LPS) activated murine B cells caused enhancement of IgG1 while inhibiting the production of IgG3 and IgG2b [35]. When the supernatant was analyzed using biochemical procedures, it was found that it contained the B cell stimulatory factor-1 which today is known as IL4 [36]. Indeed, when anti- IL4 antibodies were added to these cultures, this enhancing effect was abrogated [36]. Later, Coffman et al. observed that LPS stimulated murine splenic B cells in culture produced elevated levels of IgG1, IgG2a, IgG2b, IgM but no IgE [37]. However, when IL4 was added to the cultures of splenic B cell, IgE was produced along with the other isotypes mentioned above showing that IL4 was responsible for the production of IgE [37]. When IL5 was added to the LPS stimulated B-cell cultures, there was a significant increase in the production of IgA and it was markedly increased when the combination of IL4 and IL5 were added.

Soon after the discovery by Mosmann et al. [38] that T helper cells can be of 2 types; namely Th1 and Th2, immunologists began the tedious process of functionally characterizing the roles of these cells. With the use of mouse T helper clones, scientists were able to decipher the functions of the cytokines secreted by these T cell clones. Coffman et al. performed in vitro reconstitution experiments in which they used Th1 and Th2 clones to show how T cell can help B cells produce various isotypes [39]. The major cytokines produced by Th1 clones are IL2 and IFN-γ while Th2 clones produced IL4 and IL5. Studies revealed that when Th2 clones were stimulated in 7-day culture with mouse B cells, they produced elevated levels of the IgE, IgG1, IgM and IgA. Removal of IL4 with the use of anti-IL4 antibodies, significantly blocked the IgE response while only slightly reducing the other isotype responses.

In these early studies, Coffman et al. were also able to reconstitute the Th2 response using the Th1 clones [39]. Here, an autoreactive mouse T cell clone called H66-61 Th1 cell line was used to reconstruct a Th2 type response. Irradiated H66-61 Th1 cells were placed in 7-day culture with mouse B-cells. Therefore, these irradiated T cells cannot proliferate but can provide help to B cells. Since Th1 clones secrete IFN-γ and this cytokine can inhibit the function of IL4 in culture, anti-IFN-γ was added to all cultures. Recombinant (r) IL4 and or IL5 cytokines were added to the

H66-61 Cells + B Cells + Anti-IFN-γ +	IgE	IgG1	IgM	IgA
Medium	<1	227	1590	30
r IL4	610	4160	11,100	41
r IL5	<1	1380	15,200	208
r IL4 + r IL5	333	12,300	64,300	281
D9-Sup	577	20,700	91,900	407

All additions were added on day 0 of the cell cultures.

Table 1.
The effects of recombinant (r) IL4 and IL5 on H66-61-stimulated B cell cultures rIL4 was added at a concentration of 500 U/ml, rIL5 at 5 U/ml, D9 supernatant at 3%, anti-IFN- at 5 g/ml.

cultures yielding the isotypes as shown in **Table 1**. The results demonstrated that Th1 clone was able to provide help to the B-cells for the secretion of the isotypes that are characteristics of a Th2 response. The similarity in isotype production was observed when supernatant from a Th2 clone (D9-sup) was added to B cell cultures. Furthermore, these results showed that IL4 triggered a significant increase in the isotypes IgM, IgG1 and especially IgE. The addition of IL5 to the cultures showed a significant increase in IgA but not IgE. Previously, Sanderson et al. in 1985 used a bone marrow culture system to show that a cytokine from a specific T cell clone that is not IL2 or IL3 is an eosinophil differentiating factor [40]. Molecular cloning and genetic characterization revealed that this factor is indeed IL5 which is a growth factor for eosinophils [41, 42]. These early in vitro studies revealed that Th2 cells and their cytokines (mainly IL4 and IL5) played a prominent role in allergic responses.

3. Murine models of parasitic infection, allergy and asthma helped to demonstrate the in vivo functions of the allergic cytokines -IL4 and IL5

The role of IL4 and IL5 was further defined in experimental models using rodents infected with the nematode *Nippostrongylus brasiliensis* (Nb) larvae [43, 44]. Nb larvae, upon infection in mice pass through the lung where they molt during the first few days triggering an immune response with blood and lung eosinophilia and elevation of IgE antibodies. Coffman et al. performed an elegant study with the use of monoclonal antibodies (mAb) to IL4 and IL5 to functionally characterize the role of these cytokines in vivo [43]. BALB/c mice were injected subcutaneously (SC) with 750 third stage Nb larvae. On the same day, they were treated with 2 mg per mouse of an anti-IL5 (TRFK-5) mAb. Another infected group received 10 mg/mouse of an anti-IL4 (11B11) mAb instead of TRFK-5 mAb. Nb infected BALB/c mice showed a 25- to 100-fold increase in total IgE levels and a 4- to 8-fold increase in eosinophils. However, the group that was treated with anti-IL5 showed no increase in blood and lung tissue eosinophils but made the normal increases in serum IgE as expected from the infection. This inhibition of eosinophils by TRFK-5 also blocked the development of eosinophils from the progenitors in the bone marrow [44]. The infected group that was treated with 11B11 made significantly reduced levels of total serum IgE (**Table 2**) but made elevated levels of eosinophils as characteristic of an Nb-infected mouse. The inability of TRFK-5 to block the IgE response was consistent with previous in vitro work by Coffman et al. [39]. This was the first in vivo model to demonstrate the

Treatment	Total serum IgE (μg/ml) on days		
	-7	11	14
No antibody	0.87 (0.43)	32.4 (9.7)	31.1 (11.2)
Anti-IL-5	0.53 (0.34)	34.3 (19.9)	34.9 (20)
Anti-IL-4	1.85 (0.83)	2.5 (1.6)	3.5 (2.4)
IgG1 Control	1.15 (0.23)	12.0 (6.7)	24.8 (7.7)

Table 2.
Total serum IgE in BALB/c mice after subcutaneous injection of Nippostrongylus brasiliensis.

ability of antibodies to IL5 to block eosinophilia. This seminal study on the independent regulation of IgE and eosinophils was later confirmed by others using mouse models of allergy, asthma and allergic aspergillosis [45, 46].

Savelkoul et al. further clarified the necessity of IL4 for an IgE response from the in vivo model of inflammation using Nb infected SJA/9 mice [47]. SJA/9 mice genetically have an SJL background (H-2^s) and bear the BALB/c H chain allotype [Ig^a] [48]. They are unable to mount IgE responses to allergenic substances and helminthic parasites [48]. When the T cells of Nb- infected SJA/9 mice were placed in culture with the mitogen concanavalin A, IL4 was produced in the supernatant. Furthermore, when B cells from Nb infected SJA/9 mice were placed in culture with IL4 and LPS, IgE was produced. Similarly, the administration of rIL4 to Nb infected SJA/9 mice resulted in IgE production as they made significant levels of serum IgE which was comparable to strains that are normal IgE responders. These Nb infected mice made eosinophils that were blocked when these mice were treated with anti-IL5. Thus, IgE defect was restored by administration of IL4 to these SJA/9 mice. This study further confirmed that the contribution of IgE and eosinophil to immune responses are controlled independently by IL4 and IL5 respectively. Today, it is known that IL4 is a switch factor for the production of IgE [49] and IL5 does not act on human B cells but is the major cytokine responsible for eosinophil maturation, differentiation and survival [19].

4. How strain variations in mice influenced the allergic response to the allergenic substance ovalbumin (OVA)

A study was done to examine the allergic response from various strains of mice that were classified by the quantity of allergic antibodies (lgE) they produced after immunization with the allergenic substance- ovalbumin (OVA) [50]. These classifications were termed "high," "low," and "non" responders according to the levels of IgE mice produce upon stimulation with allergens. Therefore, experiments were performed on SJA/9, BALB/c, C57BL/6 and 129SvEv mice to examine their abilities to make an allergic response. Except for the IgE non responder strain SJA/9, all strains are capable of mounting IgE responses to allergenic substances. The aim of this study was to understand the genetics of these strains of mice with respect to IgE production to gain an understanding of the immunogenicity of individuals with a genetic predisposition to allergy and asthma.

Mice were immunized by intraperitoneal (IP) injection with 1O μg OVA in aluminum hydroxide (OVA/AL) on day O followed by exposure to a 1% aerosolized OVA which was done on day 27. Using this experimental protocol, OVA-specific lgE was elevated in all groups except in the SJA/9 strain in which it was undetectable (**Figure 1**).

It was hypothesized that this lack of lgE secretion in SJA/9 mice is due to a mechanism which is similar to that which is responsible for the nonallergic state in some individuals. OVA specific IgE peaked in all IgE responsive groups at about day 8 after the challenge with aerosolized OVA. The largest amount of lgE was seen in the 129SvEv mice while the lowest detectable amount was from the C57BL/6. After the peak response, OVA specific-lgE remained detectable in the last collection of serum which was on day 100.

Eosinophils in the blood were quantified after the first inhalation of aerosolized OVA (data not shown). All mice had elevated levels of blood eosinophils 5 days after this inhalation. Although, there were no lgE in the blood of SJA/9, this group had the highest level of blood eosinophils. Two weeks after the aerosol challenge, eosinophils remained significantly elevated in the 129/SvEv group when compared to the others.

At this point, it was necessary to examine the cytokine profile in the lung of each strain of mice. Thus, on day 150, all mice were rechallenged with a 1% aerosolized OVA and their lung cytokines assessed 4 days after this tertiary challenge. **Table 3** shows that despite the high levels of OVA-specific lgE from the 129/SvEv group, IL4 was very low in this group. OVA-specific lgE and IL4 were undetectable in SJA/9 mice. The highest level of IL4 was seen in BALB/c mice with 888 ± 301 ng/ml in the lung

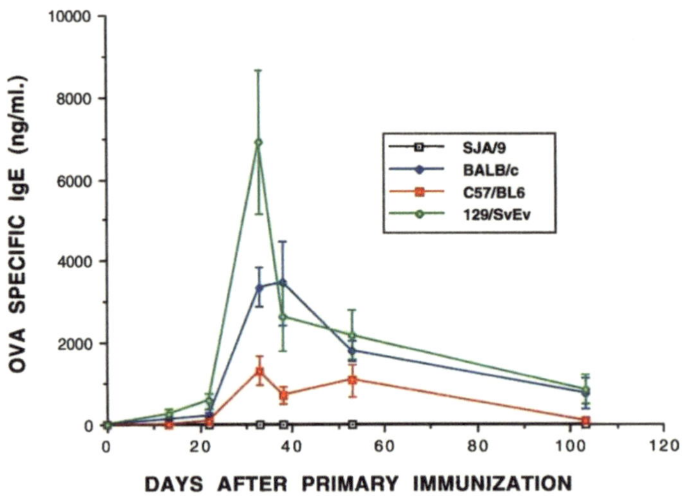

Figure 1.
IgE responses from various strains of mice after exposure to OVA.

Strain	IL3 (ng/ml)	IL4 (pg/ml)	IL5 (ng/ml)	IFN-γ (ng/ml)
SJA/9	<0.156	<1.56	1.11 ± 0.41	<0.156
C57/BL9	<0.156	70 ± 24	3.09 ± 1.00	<0.156
BALB/c	0.556 ± 0.0830	888 ± 301	8.94 ± 2.09	<0.156
129/SvEv	<0.156	34 ± 10	3.56 ± 1.24	<0.156

All mice received 10 ug OVA/AL IP on day 0 and 1% aerosolized OVA for 20 minutes on day 27 and day 150. In vitro restimulation of unseparated lung cells were done on day 154.

Table 3.
Lung cytokines from OVA immunized strains of mice.

of these mice. IFN-γ was not detected in any of the groups demonstrating that the immune response was not a Th1 type response. IL3 was detected in the BALB/c mice but not in the other groups.

The result of this experiment confirms previous studies that IL4 is a necessary cytokine for the production of IgE [47]. That is, SJA/9 mice did not produce detectable levels of IgE and did not produce any IL4 after the OVA specific in vitro restimulation of homogenized lung cells. This study also shows that IL4 is necessary but not fully responsible for the production of IgE since the highest levels of IgE came from the 129SvEv mice even though IL4 in this group was very low compared to the BALB/c group. Presently, it is known that IL13 also plays a role in the production of IgE [51]. Low levels of IL5 were seen in the SJA/9 mice when compared to the BALB/c mice (1.11 ± 0.41 vs. 8.94 ± 2.09 respectively). However, the eosinophils in the SJA/9 strains were highest when compared to the other groups. Despite the absence of IL4 and IgE from the SJA/9 strain, a Th2 response (eosinophilia and Th2 cytokines) was seen in this group. The lack of IFN-γ from all the strains revealed that these animals were not responding with a Th 1 type response, instead they are capable of producing an allergic type of response even in the SJA/9 strain that lacked detectable IgE and IL4. The level of the response from each strain may represent the atopic state of a particular strain. The SJA/9 strain represents the low responders while the 129/SvEv with their high levels of IgE may be mice which can be comparable to atopic individuals.

5. The complex role of the cytokines and inflammatory mediators in severe eosinophilic asthma

5.1 Damaged epithelial cells release alarmins to initiate the innate immune response

Numerous studies have been performed which have recognized the major regulatory mechanisms in allergic airway diseases [4, 52, 53]. There are many multifactorial events that are necessary for a non-allergic individual to develop allergic airway disease such as severe eosinophilic asthma (**Figure 2**). It begins with damaged lung epithelial cells after an atopic individual is exposed to aeroallergens such as pollen and/or environmental irritants such as tobacco smoke [54]. The damaged epithelium secretes the alarmins -IL33, IL25 and TSLP [55, 56]. These cytokines can cause a shift in the immune response towards an allergic phenotype with pathological consequences related to airway allergic disease [55]. For example, in a mouse model of asthma, mice treated intranasally with IL25, developed epithelial cell hyperplasia, mucus hyper-secretion and bronchial hyperreactivity [57]. Indeed, severe asthmatic patients with fixed airflow limitation show an increase in IL25 [58]. Others have shown that the level of circulating fibrocytes (progenitor cells that enter the circulation and inflame the bronchial epithelium) bearing the receptor for IL25 correlates with the severity of asthma [59].

IL33 is a member of the IL1 family which participates in the polarization of the immune response towards a T2 type inflammation. It is expressed not only by epithelial cells but also by vascular endothelia cells. Atopic patients chronically exposed to environmental pollutants or allergens containing serine proteases will show an early increase in IL33 from their damaged epithelial cells. This cytokine is present in the bronchoalveolar lavage and airway smooth muscles, and they activate dendritic

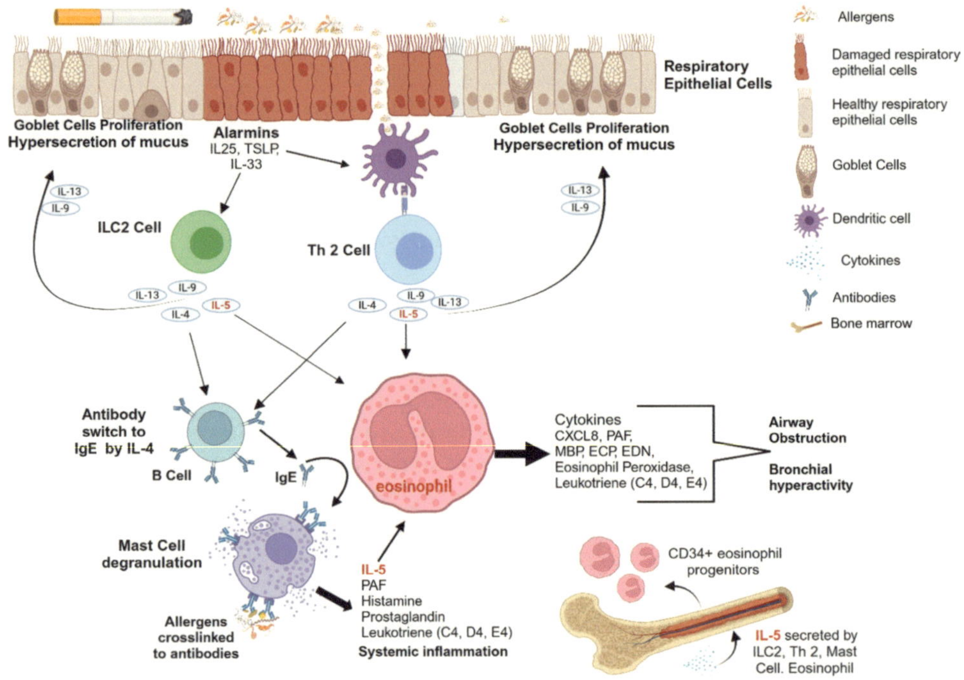

Figure 2.
The interaction of the alarmins with the T2 cytokines and the prolongation of eosinophilia from damaged epithelial cells of the airways (image created with BioRender.com).

cells - the major antigen presenting cells [60]. Thus, the expression of IL33 in humans can lead to atopic diseases with elevated levels of IgE, hyper eosinophilia and asthma.

The thymic stromal lymphopoietin (TSLP) is another cytokine that is secreted by the damaged epithelial cell in response to proteases [61, 62]. TSLP is a member of the IL2 cytokines family, and its gene can be found on the human chromosome at 5q22.1 which is close to the cluster of cytokines- IL4, 5 and 13 located at 5q3185 [63]. TSLP is also expressed in lung fibroblast, and smooth muscle. Its receptor is expressed on innate lymphoid cell type 2 (ILC2), dendritic cells, T cells, B cells, mast cells, basophils, monocytes and eosinophils [61]. It is involved in dendritic cells maturation and the skewing of T helper cells to a Th2 phenotype particularly during an allergic response [64]. Indeed, TSLP's mRNA and protein are elevated in asthmatic patients and correlate with airway hyperresponsiveness regardless of the levels of eosinophilia and T2 inflammation [52, 65].

Collectively, the alarmins work together to activate the ILC2 cell during the innate phase of the allergic response by contributing to the initiation of the inflammatory response. ILC2 cells are the early producers of several T2 cytokines including IL4, IL5, IL9, IL13 [66]. The ILCs which arise from the common lymphoid progenitor are closely related to the Natural Killer (NK) cells. They reside in peripheral tissues and are categorized into 3 groups namely 1, 2 and 3 according to the cytokines they produce and their surface characteristics [67].

It was found that when ILC cells were stimulated with IL25 and IL33, the neuro-peptide receptor Nmur1 was expressed preferentially by ILC2 cells. Furthermore, when neuromedin U (NMU), the ligand for Nmur1 was co administered with IL25, they amplified the allergic inflammation with increases in eosinophils in the lung and broncho alveolar lavage [68]. TSLP and to a lesser extent IL25 and IL33 from epithelial cells causes the release of IL5 from ILC2 cells. Also, studies have shown that when TSLP was added to IL33-stimulated ILC2 human cells, the production of IL4, IL5 and IL13 was enhanced along with increase expression of the transcription factor GATA3 [69]. This transcription is required for the expression of IL5 from Th2 cells [69]. IL13 produced by ILC2 cells is necessary for the migration of dendritic cells to the draining lymph nodes where they induce naïve T cells to become Th2 cells during the process of T cell activation. TSLP stimulated dendritic cells has been shown to lead to the production of chemokines CCL17 and CCL21 and ultimately to the priming of Th2 cells [64]. In chronic conditions, TSLP downregulates the development of Tregs while maintaining the Th2 type inflammation [64]. Indeed, TSLP is increased in the airway walls of patients with severe asthma. Thus, the ILC2 cell, due to its early secretion of cytokines, participates in the innate phase and is necessary for the adaptive phase of the allergic response as naïve T cells differentiate into effector Th2 cells [70, 71].

IL3, IL5 and GM-CSF participate in the development of eosinophils however, IL5 is the major cytokine for its development, and it is at center stage in patients with severe eosinophilic asthma [31]. Though the main cellular sources of IL5 are Th2 and ILC2 cells, it is also secreted by other cells such as mast cells, basophils, NKT cells and eosinophils themselves pointing to the increase in eosinophils as largely due to the many sources of IL5 [26, 72–74]. Meanwhile, the damaged epithelial cells also secrete chemokines CCL5 (RANTES) and CCL11 (eotaxin-1) that can bind to a receptor called CCR3. Also, IL4 and IL13 can stimulate epithelial cells in the lungs to produce eotaxins [75]. The CCR3 receptor is expressed on Th2 cells, macrophages, eosinophils, basophils and mast cells [31, 76]. While eotaxin-1 is required for the initial steps in the inflammatory response, eotaxin-2 and eotaxin-3 participate in the prolongation of eosinophil survival [31]. Thus, there will be an influx of these cells from the blood to the respiratory tract which contributes to the obstruction of the airways.

5.2 Th2 type allergic response is responsible for the adaptive phase and participates in the prolongation of the chronic inflammation in severe eosinophilic asthma

After the initial phase of the allergic response, Th2 cells with the series of cytokines they produce which are mainly IL4, IL5, and IL13 play a prominent role in propagating the chronic inflammation seen in severe eosinophilic asthma. IL4, a switch factor for IgE, is largely responsible for the increase in allergic antibodies. IgE attaches to mast cells via the high affinity Fc epsilon receptor. If crosslinking of antigen occurs via the fragment antigen-binding (FAB) region, then the mast cell becomes degranulated as shown in **Figure 2** with the release of inflammatory mediators such as histamine, chemotactic factors, cytokines, metabolites of arachidonic acid. These mediators act on vasculature, goblet cells, smooth muscles and inflammatory cells in the airways to bring about bronchoconstriction [77]. IL4 also promotes the commitment for the differentiation of naïve T cells to Th2 cells. The IL4 receptor activates STAT6 from the naïve T cell which promotes the expression of the transcription factor -GATA3. The B lymphocyte-induced maturation protein-1 (Blimp-1) enhances the GATA3 expression in T helper cells causing them to differentiate to Th2 cells with amplification of the inflammatory allergic response in atopic individuals exposed to aeroallergens [78]. Therefore, IL4 with its ability to cause naïve T cells to commit to a Th2 pathway, plays a prominent role in the prolonged elevation of IL5 in severe eosinophilic asthma. Epithelial cell activation occurs due to the presence of IL-5, IL-13, and periostin, (a protein upregulated by IL-13) which also causes the biomarker FeNO for a Th2 inflammation to be expressed [79]. Together, IL13 and IL9 have a role in bronchial hyperreactivity and the remodeling of the airway epithelium by causing epithelial cells to differentiate into goblet cells [4]. The increase in goblet cells can lead to a hyper secretion of mucus in an asthmatic individual [4, 80, 81].

The high levels of IL5, particularly in the bronchial tracts, in patients with severe eosinophilic asthma can hinder the pro-apoptotic effect from the treatment with corticosteroids [82]. This refractory state is defined as severe T2-high eosinophilic asthma in which eosinophils accumulate and proliferate throughout the airways. The IL5 receptor alpha chain is expressed on eosinophils, airway epithelial cells and lung fibroblast [78, 83]. The elevated presence of IL5 and eosinophils can lead to the development of co-morbidities such as chronic rhinosinusitis and nasal polyps due to the continuous production and survival of eosinophils in the bronchial tracts [79]. These patients experience frequent exacerbation of their allergic phenotype and difficulty controlling their respiratory conditions. The unraveling of the function of Th2 cytokines, particularly IL5, in maintaining the elevated levels of eosinophils has aroused the interest of researchers to explore the use of biological markers for therapeutic intervention in severe eosinophilic asthma [84, 85]. This development of biologics can be the key to control severe eosinophilic asthma when it is uncontrollable with the use of corticosteroids due to the high levels of IL-5.

6. The use of biologics for the treatment of eosinophilic asthma

The first published report that antibodies to IL5 can inhibit eosinophils in vivo was done using a mouse model of *Nippostrongylus brasiliensis* infected parasitized mice in 1989 [43]. Later scientists used a monkey model of asthma and a mouse model of pulmonary inflammation to also demonstrate the inhibitory effect of anti-IL5 on eosinophils [86, 87]. These preclinical studies paved the way for the use of anti-IL5 biologicals in the treatment of severe eosinophilic asthma. Over the last decade, biologics that target cytokines and cytokine receptors, have been developed to be used as an adjuvant therapy in the management of severe eosinophilic asthma [88–91]. Several clinical trials have evaluated the efficacy of anti-IL5 or anti-IL5 receptor antibodies in patients with asthma [92, 93]. These biologics are: Mepolizumab, Reslizumab and Benralizumab.

Mepolizumab is a humanized mAb (IgG1 k type), originated by binding anti human IL5 antigen recognition sites from murine origins into a human IgG1 heavy chain [94]. It has a high affinity in binding free IL-5 (a 134 amino acid dimeric glycoprotein with 4 helix bundle mortif that has a 52-KDa homodimer) resulting in IL-5 inability to bind to the receptor IL5Rα (**Figure 3**) [94, 95]. This binding causes a reduction of eosinophils in both the blood and airways [96]. Its very specific binding ability may explain the lack of relatively significant side effects of Mepolizumab as it does not seem to interfere with the biological activities of other cytokines [94]. However, early studies with Mepolizumab showed mixed response from clinical trials conducted in several asthmatic patients' population where there was documented reduction in circulating eosinophils without much significant clinical response in the severity of the disease [92, 97]. These early investigations included a small population study that was conducted on difficult to treat asthmatic patients whose treatment included high dose ICS and/or oral corticosteroid (OCS). This study also showed a similar outcome in reduction of blood eosinophils with little effect on the clinical outcome, except for a small improvement in lung FEV1 (forced expiratory volume in 1 second) function [98]. Many of these early studies were done in which a specific

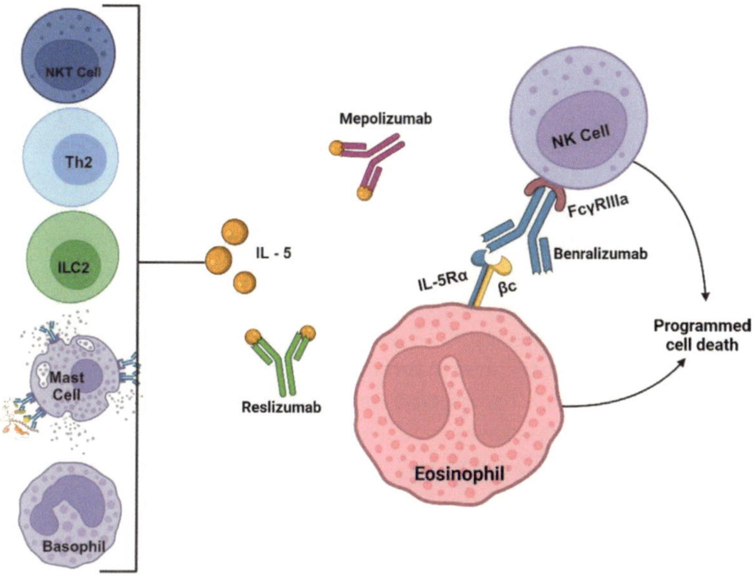

Figure 3.
The mechanisms of action of reslizumab, mepolizumab and benralizumab on eosinophils. Reslizumab and mepolizumab use different idiotypic regions to bind to the IL5 molecule. The FAB region of Benralizumab attaches to the IL5 receptor on the eosinophil and the Benralizumab's Fc region attaches to the Fcγ receptor as shown on the NK cell to induce ADCC. The sources of IL5 are also shown (image created with BioRender.com).

participant group consisted of various asthma phenotypes ranging from mild to moderate chronic asthma. Despite the reduction of eosinophils, the quality of life for these patients was not improved with respect to asthma exacerbation rates [93].

Eventually, investigators examined patients suffering solely from severe chronic asthma [99]. This small study involved patients with bronchial eosinophilia who were not responsive to treatment with corticosteroids. The result of this study showed reduction not only in eosinophil levels but also in asthma exacerbations after treatment with Mepolizumab. Later, a 52-weeks study termed; the DREAM (Dose Ranging Efficacy And safety with Mepolizumab in severe asthma) study was conducted as one of the largest asthma studies (621 participants) to examine the effect of Mepolizumab in participants with severe asthma [100]. The study had strict criteria that required at least 2 exacerbation which included the use of OCS or a visit to an emergency room or hospitalization and signs of eosinophilic inflammation (either sputum eosinophils >3%, peripheral blood eosinophils >300 x 10^6/L, FeNO>50 ppb or loss of asthma control after <25% reduction in either ICS or OCS dose). Participants received 13 infusions of either 75, 250 or 750 mg of intravenous (IV) mepolizumab. Results showed all three doses significantly reduced asthma exacerbation equally and reduced both blood and sputum eosinophils [100].

Mepolizumab as Adjunctive Therapy in Patients with Severe Asthma (MENSA) was a study of 576 asthmatic patients over 52 weeks who were treated with ICS with or without OCS [101]. They were randomized to receive either 75 or 100 mg mepolizumab SC every 4 weeks or a placebo. The inclusion criteria were asthmatic with at least 2 exacerbations requiring systemic corticosteroids the previous year with evidence of eosinophilic inflammation (eosinophil count 150 cells/uL at screening or above 300 cells/μL at some point in the previous year). Results showed a 47 and 53% respectively in IV and SC mepolizumab associated reduction in asthma exacerbations [101].

Mechanistically, investigators have shown that after treatment with Mepolizumab, there is a decrease in PD-1 expression on Tregs hereby allowing this subset of cells to perform its immunomodulatory duty [102]. TGF-β is also reduced after severe asthmatics with eosinophilia are treated with Mepolizumab. This cytokine is secreted by many cells in the respiratory tract but is mainly liberated by eosinophils [103]. It is believed to play a role in the differentiation of fibroblast to myofibroblasts which participates in airway remodeling. Thus, with the treatment of severe asthmatics with Mepolizumab, there was a reduced expression of some extracellular matrix proteins and consequently the reduction of airway remodeling [31, 102]. Corticosteroids have been shown to be ineffective in reducing airway remodeling in patients with chronic asthma particularly those with severe eosinophilic asthma. Therefore, Mepolizumab is a necessary add-on therapeutic for the inhibition of fibrosis and airway remodeling of individuals with severe eosinophilic asthma which accounted for approximately 5% of all asthmatics [14, 31]. This treatment also reduces the severity of exacerbation even in patients with comorbidity such as bronchiectasis [104]. The FDA and the European Medicines Agency both eventually approved Mepolizumab as an adjuvant treatment for severe eosinophilic asthma [93].

Reslizumab, another anti-IL5 mAb showed significant improvement in lung function in a study (P = 0.002 vs. placebo) with trend towards improved asthma score and reduction in sputum eosinophils [96]. It is an IL-5 neutralizing IgG4K mAb, that is currently approved for adjunct therapy for adults with severe eosinophilic asthma [91]. Data from the BREATH phase 111 clinical trial which involved three double -blinded studies in patients 12–75 year with eosinophilic asthma not controlled on an ICS used reslizumab 3 mg/kg once every 4 weeks for 52 weeks. The results in various subgroups showed a significant reduction in asthma exacerbation frequencies, lung function and improved quality of life [105]. Ibrahim et al., explored the clinical efficacy of Reslizumab in patients with inadequately controlled asthma, elevated blood eosinophils, taking high dose ICS, a second controller with at least 4 exacerbations and one hospitalization [106]. The results were statistically significant through the use of a validated asthma control questionnaire. Of note, patients had a decrease in maintenance steroid usage while taking Reslizumab [106]. In comparison of severity, patients with late-onset eosinophilic asthma were noted to have a greater response to Reslizumab in reductions of exacerbation and improvement to lung function than those with early-onset asthma [91, 107].

Benralizumab, is an anti-IL5-receptor cytolytic mAb that binds directly to the IL-5 receptors on eosinophils thus enabling the immune system to remove them [108]. It is a humanized IgG1k, afucosylated mAb, (lacking oligosaccharides in the Fc region) which works by inducing apoptosis in target cells via antibody-dependent cellular cytotoxicity (ADCC) (**Figure 3**). In comparison to the other anti -IL-5 biologics, it has the most efficiency in the depletion of eosinophil in peripheral blood [96]. Others have observed clinically and statistically significant reduction in asthma exacerbations with the addition of Benralizumab with current treatment protocols. Some patients were able to discontinue systemic steroid therapy and became exacerbation-free by this adjunct therapy [108, 109]. However, studies have shown bronchial eosinophils remained after treatment with Benralizumab [85]. Investigators have shown that there exists a subset of lung-resident eosinophils with regulatory functions which are different from the inflammatory eosinophils that participate in the Th2 responses [110–112]. These lung resident homeostatic eosinophils are IL5 independent while the inflammatory eosinophils are IL5 dependent [107]. Indeed, IL5 deficient mice have reduced level of basal eosinophils and are unable to produce an eosinophilic inflammation as in the context of the Th2 response [110]. Therefore, the eosinophils in the bronchial tree that remained after treatment with anti-IL5 biologics may be the protective homeostasis eosinophils as those remaining may be responsible for the lack of increased risk of infection after treatment [113]. Overall, the therapeutic effect of anti-IL5 demonstrates that IL5 is the major cytokine responsible for the activation and survival of eosinophils [114]. Presently, the GINA recommendations for anti IL5 therapy are on the final Stepwise (step 5) approach to the management of severe asthma [21].

Beside targeting IL5 and its receptor for the treatment of severe eosinophilic asthma, other T2 cytokines have been targeted successfully and are currently approved. Dupilumab is a fully human mAb that blocks the alpha receptor subunit of IL-4, blocking both IL-4 and IL-13 since they share a common subunit [115]. The first clinical trial involved 52 patients with severe eosinophil asthma who were given dupilumab at a dose of 300 mg SC while 52 with similar baseline characteristic were given a placebo. The results showed that only 6% of participants from the dupilumab group continued to have asthma exacerbation versus 44% in the placebo group. This study was a 12-week provocative method where long-acting β2 agonist (LABA) was discontinued at week 4 and ICS at weeks 6–9. The results showed an 87% reduction in asthma exacerbation, improved lung function and Th2 inflammatory markers when compared to the placebo [116]. Several other studies have concluded that Dupilumab was effective in decreasing asthma exacerbation, improving lung function and quality of life in patients with asthma [117, 118].

Omalizumab, an anti-IgE mAb, downregulates IgE receptors by inhibiting IgE binding to mast cells, dendritic cells and basophils which results in the inhibition of IgE mediated inflammation. Consequently, Omalizumab treatment decreased eosinophils and multiple inflammatory mediators. It is one of the biologics currently being utilized for the treatment of moderate to severe allergic asthma with a positive treatment response [119].

Tezepelumab is a human mAb that binds to TSLP. In a randomized, double blind, placebo-controlled 52 weeks trial in patients with uncontrolled asthma who were on LABA and medium to high dose ICS, 3 doses of Tezepelumab were compared to placebo [31]. Asthma exacerbation rates were significantly reduced irrespective of the baseline eosinophil blood count or despite the dose (low, medium, or high) given. However, health related quality of life was only noted to be improved in the high dose group [31]. It has been FDA approved for children ages 12 years and older and adults with severe eosinophilic asthma.

7. Concluding remarks

The use of mAb to treat severe eosinophilic asthma has been effective as observed in clinical trials and real-world clinical efficacy studies [101–103, 120–121]. Biologic therapy as an adjunct treatment has decreased the number of asthma exacerbations, reported symptom days, and improved lung function. Across the studies these improvements have been particularly notable in those with the highest blood eosinophil counts when anti-IL5 biologics were compared to omalizumab and dupilumab [118, 122–124]. This treatment works for asthmatics with severe eosinophilia [118]. However, the benefits of biologics in moderate asthma are still an ongoing area of study.

The main limitations of biologics in asthma treatments are their high cost and the tedious ongoing research into the pathogenesis of the subtypes of severe asthma [107]. The variations in endotypes pose challenges to its application in various patient populations. The utilization of biomarkers such as IgE, eosinophil count and FeNO have been shown to be beneficial for identification of endotypes especially for severe eosinophil asthmatic patients at increased risk of exacerbations [89, 119, 125, 126]. However, their identification and treatment can also be challenging due to the varying amounts of overlap of eosinophilic asthma with other endotypes particularly T2 and allergic asthma. Biomarkers such as eosinophil counts can be misleading because environmental factors can cause natural fluctuation in baseline count as observed in some healthy individuals. For example, healthy individuals exposed to tobacco smoke have a significantly higher median eosinophil count compared to nonsmokers making it difficult to determine the necessity for the use of biologics as add on in treatment [17]. Also, race should be considered as a factor when implementing treatment for vulnerable demographics. African Americans are at a higher risk for morbidity and mortality from severe asthma and studies show that those on ICS exhibit higher levels of eosinophilic inflammation than their white counterparts [127]. Finally, early identification of at-risk individuals can be instrumental in the prevention and treatment of severe eosinophilic asthma as it would potentially reduce the need for healthcare resources as medicine becomes more personalized.

Acknowledgements

This research was supported in part by HCA Healthcare and/or an HCA Healthcare affiliated entity.

The views expressed in this publication represent those of the author(s) and do not necessarily represent the official views of HCA Healthcare or any of its affiliated entities. This project has received funding from the US National Science Foundation (NSF) Research and Innovation program under the Grant Agreement no. 2000433. The authors wish to acknowledge the contributions of Annik T. Segree and Bethnay M. Simmons in the preparation of this chapter.

Author details

Brian W.P. Seymour[1*], Ashley A. Seymour[2] and Patricia M. Gilford[3]

1 Edward Waters University, Jacksonville, Florida, USA

2 Department of Internal Medicine, The Ohio State University Wexner Medical Center, Columbus, OH, USA

3 HCA Florida Orange Park Hospital, Family Medicine Residency Program, Florida, USA

*Address all correspondence to: brian.seymour@ew.edu

References

[1] Sinyor B, Concepcion Perez L. Pathophysiology of asthma. In: StatPearls [Internet]. Treasure Island (FL): StatPearls Publishing; 2023. [Copyright in 2024]

[2] Holgate ST, Wenzel S, Postma DS, et al. Asthma. Nature Reviews. Disease Primers. 2015;**1**:15025. DOI: 10.1038/nrdp.2015.25

[3] McCracken JL, Veeranki SP, Ameredes BT, Calhoun WJ. Diagnosis and management of asthma in adults: A review. Journal of the American Medical Association. 2017;**318**(3):279-290. DOI: 10.1001/jama.2017.8372

[4] Gour N, Wills-Karp M. IL-4 and IL-13 signaling in allergic airway disease. Cytokine. 2015;**75**:68-78. DOI: 10.1016/j.cyto.2015.05.014

[5] Gans MD, Gavrilova T. Understanding the immunology of asthma: Pathophysiology, biomarkers, and treatments for asthma endotypes. Paediatric Respiratory Reviews. 2020;**36**:118-127. DOI: 10.1016/j.prrv.2019.08.002

[6] Nunes C, Pereira AM, Morais-Almeida M. Asthma costs and social impact. Asthma Research and Practice. 2017;**3**:1. DOI: 10.1186/s40733-016-0029-3

[7] Daya M, Barnes KC. African American ancestry contribution to asthma and atopic dermatitis. Annals of Allergy, Asthma and Immunology. 2019;**122**:456-462. DOI: 10.1016/j.anai.2019.02.009

[8] Bateman ED, Hurd SS, Barnes PJ, et al. Global strategy for asthma management and prevention: GINA executive summary. The European Respiratory Journal. 2008;**31**(1):143-178. DOI: 10.1183/09031936.00138707

[9] Serebrisky D, Wiznia A. Pediatric asthma: A global epidemic. Annals of Global Health. 2019;**85**(1):6. DOI: 10.5334/aogh.2416

[10] Wenzel SE. Asthma phenotypes: The evolution from clinical to molecular approaches. Nature Medicine. 2012;**18**:716-725. DOI: 10.1038/nm.2678

[11] Lötvall J, Akdis CA, Bacharier LB, et al. Asthma endotypes: A new approach to classification of disease entities within the asthma syndrome. The Journal of Allergy and Clinical Immunology. 2011;**127**(2):355-360. DOI: 10.1016/j.jaci.2010.11.037

[12] Backman H, Räisänen P, Hedman L, et al. Increased prevalence of allergic asthma from 1996 to 2006 and further to 2016-results from three population surveys. Clinical and Experimental Allergy. 2017;**47**:1426-1435. DOI: 10.1111/cea.12963

[13] Chen M, Shepard K 2nd, Ming Yang M, et al. Overlap of allergic, eosinophilic and type 2 inflammatory subtypes in moderate-to-severe asthma. Clinical and Experimental Allergy. 2021;**51**:546-555. DOI: 10.1111/cea.13790

[14] Tan LD, Bratt JM, Godor D, et al. Benralizumab: A unique IL-5 inhibitor for severe asthma. Journal of Asthma and Allergy. 2016;**9**:71-81. DOI: 10.2147/JAA.S78049

[15] Adamiec A, Cieślik M, Maczka K, et al. A systematic review and meta-analysis on absolute eosinophil counts and the risk of asthma in preschool

children with wheezing: An EAACI task force report. Pediatric Allergy and Immunology. 2024;**35**:e14078. DOI: 10.1111/pai.14078

[16] Li H, Li X. Genetic relationships between high blood eosinophil count, asthma susceptibility, and asthma severity. The Journal of Asthma. 2024;**61**:119-131. DOI: 10.1080/02770903.2023.2247490

[17] Lommatzsch M, Nair P, Virchow JC. Normal blood eosinophil counts in humans. Respiration. 2024;**103**(4):214-216. DOI: 10.1159/000537833

[18] Seymour BW, Schelegle ES, Pinkerton KE, et al. Second-hand smoke increases bronchial hyperreactivity and eosinophilia in a murine model of allergic aspergillosis. Clinical and Developmental Immunology. 2003;**10**:35-42. DOI: 10.1080/10446670310001598483

[19] Bochner BS, Gleich GJ. What targeting eosinophils has taught us about their role in diseases. The Journal of Allergy and Clinical Immunology. 2010;**126**:16-25. DOI: 10.1016/j.jaci.2010.02.026

[20] Bousquet J, Chanez P, Lacoste JY, et al. Eosinophilic inflammation in asthma. The New England Journal of Medicine. 1990;**323**:1033-1039. DOI: 10.1056/NEJM199010113231505

[21] Levy ML, Bacharier LB, Bateman E, et al. Key recommendations for primary care from the 2022 global initiative for asthma (GINA) update. NPJ Primary Care Respiratory Medicine. 2023;**33**(1):7. DOI: 10.1038/s41533-023-00330-1

[22] Agache I, Akdis CA, Akdis M, et al. EAACI biologicals guidelines-recommendations for severe asthma. Allergy. 2021;**76**:14-44. DOI: 10.1111/all.14425

[23] Tran TN, Zeiger RS, Peters SP, et al. Overlap of atopic, eosinophilic, and TH2-high asthma phenotypes in a general population with current asthma. Annals of Allergy, Asthma and Immunology. 2016;**116**:37-42. DOI: 10.1016/j.anai.2015.10.027

[24] Pavlidis S, Takahashi K, Kwong FNK, et al. "T2-high" in severe asthma related to blood eosinophil, exhaled nitric oxide and serum periostin. The European Respiratory Journal. 2019;**53**(1):1800938. DOI: 10.1183/13993003.00938-2018

[25] Del Pozo V, Bobolea I, Rial MJ, et al. Expert consensus on the use of systemic glucocorticoids for managing eosinophil-related diseases. Frontiers in Immunology. 2024;**14**:1310211. DOI: 10.3389/fimmu.2023.1310211

[26] Pelaia C, Paoletti G, Puggioni F, et al. Interleukin-5 in the pathophysiology of severe asthma. Frontiers in Physiology. 2019;**10**:1514. DOI: 10.3389/fphys.2019.01514

[27] Stirling RG, van Rensen EL, Barnes PJ, Chung KF. Interleukin-5 induces CD34(+) eosinophil progenitor mobilization and eosinophil CCR3 expression in asthma. American Journal of Respiratory and Critical Care Medicine. 2001;**164**(8 Pt. 1):1403-1409. DOI: 10.1164/ajrccm.164.8.2010002

[28] Fulkerson PC, Rothenberg ME. Targeting eosinophils in allergy, inflammation and beyond. Nature Reviews. Drug Discovery. 2013;**12**:117-129. DOI: 10.1038/nrd3838

[29] Dunican EM, Fahy JV. Asthma and corticosteroids: Time for a more precise approach to treatment. The European Respiratory Journal. 2017;**49**:1701167. DOI: 10.1183/13993003.01167-2017

[30] Agache I, Beltran J, Akdis C, et al. Efficacy and safety of treatment with

biologicals (benralizumab, dupilumab, mepolizumab, omalizumab and reslizumab) for severe eosinophilic asthma. A systematic review for the EAACI guidelines—Recommendations on the use of biologicals in severe asthma. Allergy. 2020;**75**(5):1023-1042. DOI: 10.1111/all.14221

[31] Bakakos A, Loukides S, Bakakos P. Severe eosinophilic asthma. Journal of Clinical Medicine. 2019;**8**:1375. DOI: 10.3390/jcm8091375

[32] Kay AB, Phipps S, Robinson DS. A role for eosinophils in airway remodelling in asthma. Trends in Immunology. 2004;**25**:477-482. DOI: 10.1016/j.it.2004.07.006

[33] Cho JY, Miller M, Baek KJ, et al. Inhibition of airway remodeling in IL-5-deficient mice. The Journal of Clinical Investigation. 2004;**113**:551-560. DOI: 10.1172/JCI1913

[34] Tanaka H, Komai M, Nagao K, et al. Role of interleukin-5 and eosinophils in allergen-induced airway remodeling in mice. American Journal of Respiratory Cell and Molecular Biology. 2004;**31**:62-68. DOI: 10.1165/rcmb.2003-0305OC

[35] Isakson PC, Puré E, Vitetta ES, Krammer PH. T cell-derived B cell differentiation factor(s). Effect on the isotype switch of murine B cells. The Journal of Experimental Medicine. 1982;**155**:734-748. DOI: 10.1084/jem.155.3.734

[36] Vitetta ES, Ohara J, Myers CD, et al. Serological, biochemical, and functional identity of B cell-stimulatory factor 1 and B cell differentiation factor for IgG1. The Journal of Experimental Medicine. 1985;**162**:1726-1731. DOI: 10.1084/jem.162.5.1726

[37] Coffman RL, Carty J. A T cell activity that enhances polyclonal IgE production and its inhibition by interferon-gamma. Journal of Immunology. 1986;**136**:949-954

[38] Mosmann TR, Cherwinski H, Bond MW, et al. Two types of murine helper T cell clone. I. Definition according to profiles of lymphokine activities and secreted proteins. Journal of Immunology. 1986;**136**(7):2348-2357

[39] Coffman RL, Seymour BWP, Lebman D, et al. The role of helper T cells product in mouse B cells differentiation and isotype regulation. Immunological Reviews. 1988;**102**:5-28. DOI: 10.1111/j.1600-065x.1988.tb00739.x

[40] Sanderson CJ, Warren DJ, Strath M. Identification of a lymphokine that stimulates eosinophil differentiation in vitro. Its relationship to interleukin 3, and functional properties of eosinophils produced in cultures. The Journal of Experimental Medicine. 1985;**162**(1):60-74. DOI: 10.1084/jem.162.1.60

[41] Campbell HD, Tucker WQ, Hort Y, et al. Molecular cloning, nucleotide sequence, and expression of the gene encoding human eosinophil differentiation factor (interleukin 5). Proceedings of the National Academy of Sciences of the United States of America. 1987;**84**(19):6629-6633. DOI: 10.1073/pnas.84.19.6629

[42] Clutterbuck E, Shields JG, Gordon J, et al. Recombinant human interleukin 5 is an eosinophil differentiation factor but has no activity in standard human B cell growth factor assay. European Journal of Immunology. 1987;**17**:1743-1750. DOI: 10.1002/eji.1830171210

[43] Coffman RL, Seymour BW, Hudak S, et al. Antibody to interleukin-5 inhibits helminth-induced eosinophilia in mice. Science. 1989;**245**:308-310. DOI: 10.1126/science.2787531

[44] Rennick DM, Thompson-Snipes L, Coffman RL, et al. In vivo administration of antibody to interleukin-5 inhibits increased generation of eosinophils and their progenitors in bone marrow of parasitized mice. Blood. 1990;**76**:312-316

[45] Foster PS, Hogan SP, Ramsay AJ, et al. Interleukin 5 deficiency abolishes eosinophilia, airways hyperreactivity, and lung damage in a mouse asthma model. The Journal of Experimental Medicine. 1996;**183**(1):195-201. DOI: 10.1084/jem.183.1.195

[46] Kurup VP, Choi H, Murali PS, Coffman RL. IgE and eosinophil regulation in a murine model of allergic aspergillosis. Journal of Leukocyte Biology. 1994;**56**(5):593-598. DOI: 10.1002/jlb.56.5.593

[47] Savelkoul HFJ, Seymour BWP, Sullivan L, Coffman RL. IL-4 can correct the defective Ig-E production of SJA/9 mice. Journal of Immunology. 1991;**146**:1801-1805

[48] Herzenberg LA, Okumura K, Cantor H, et al. T-cell regulation of antibody responses: Demonstration of allotype-specific helper T cells and their specific removal by suppressor T cells. The Journal of Experimental Medicine. 1976;**144**(2):330-344. DOI: 10.1084/jem.144.2.330

[49] Severinson E. Identification of the IgG1 induction factor (interleukin 4). Frontiers in Immunology. 2014;**5**:628. DOI: 10.3389/fimmu.2014.00628

[50] Seymour BWP. The effect of environmental tobacco smoke on murine models of allergy [thesis]. Davis: University of California; 1996

[51] Imraish A, Abu-Thiab T, Zihlif M. IL-13 and FOXO3 genes polymorphisms regulate IgE levels in asthmatic patients. Biomedical Reports. 2021;**14**(6):55. DOI: 10.3892/br.2021.1431

[52] Soumelis V, Reche PA, Kanzler H, et al. Human epithelial cells trigger dendritic cell mediated allergic inflammation by producing TSLP. Nature Immunology. 2002;**3**(7):673-680. DOI: 10.1038/ni805

[53] Oboki K, Nakae S, Matsumoto K, Saito H. IL-33 and airway inflammation. Allergy, Asthma and Immunology Research. 2011;**3**(2):81-88. DOI: 10.4168/aair.2011.3.2.81

[54] Shrestha SK, Katelaris C, Dharmage SC, et al. High ambient levels of grass, weed and other pollen are associated with asthma admissions in children and adolescents: A large 5-year case-crossover study. Clinical and Experimental Allergy. 2018;**48**:1421-1428. DOI: 10.1111/cea.13225

[55] Gauvreau GM, Bergeron C, Boulet L-P, et al. Sounding the alarmins-the role of alarmin cytokines in asthma. Allergy. 2023;**78**(2):402-417. DOI: 10.1111/all.15609

[56] Bradding P, Porsbjerg C, Côté A, et al. Airway hyperresponsiveness in asthma: The role of the epithelium. The Journal of Allergy and Clinical Immunology. 2024;**153**(5):1181-1193. DOI: 10.1016/j.jaci.2024.02.011

[57] Hurst SD, Muchamuel T, Gorman DM, et al. New IL-17 family members promote Th1 or Th2 responses in the lung: In vivo function of the novel cytokine IL-25. Journal of Immunology. 2002;**169**:443-453. DOI: 10.4049/jimmunol.169.1.443

[58] Yao X, Liu X, Wang X, Zhang L. IL-25R+ circulating fibrocytes are increased in asthma and correlate with fixed airflow limitation. The Clinical

Respiratory Journal. 2021;**15**(11):1248-1256. DOI: 10.1111/crj.13433

[59] Yao X, Chen Q, Wang X, et al. IL-25 induces airway remodeling in asthma by orchestrating the phenotypic changes of epithelial cell and fibrocyte. Respiratory Research. 2023;**24**(1):212. DOI: 10.1186/s12931-023-02509-z

[60] Besnard A-G, Togbe D, Guillou N, et al. IL-33-activated dendritic cells are critical for allergic airway inflammation. European Journal of Immunology. 2011;**41**(6):1675-1686. DOI: 10.1002/eji.201041033

[61] Kouzaki H, O'Grady SM, Lawrence CB, Kita H. Proteases induce production of thymic stromal lymphopoietin by airway epithelial cells through protease-activated receptor-2. Journal of Immunology. 2009;**183**(2):1427-1434. DOI: 10.4049/jimmunol.0900904

[62] Theofani E, Tsitsopoulou A, Morianos I, Semitekolou M. Severe asthmatic responses: The impact of TSLP. International Journal of Molecular Sciences. 2023;**24**(8):7581. DOI: 10.3390/ijms24087581

[63] He R, Geha RS. Thymic stromal lymphopoietin. Annals of the New York Academy of Sciences. 2010;**1183**:13-24. DOI: 10.1111/j.1749-6632.2009.05128.x

[64] Cianferoni A, Spergel J. The importance of TSLP in allergic disease and its role as a potential therapeutic target. Expert Review of Clinical Immunology. 2014;**10**(11):1463-1474. DOI: 10.1586/1744666X.2014.967684

[65] Andreasson LM, Dyhre-Petersen N, Hvidtfeldt M, et al. Airway hyperresponsiveness correlates with airway TSLP in asthma independent of eosinophilic inflammation. The Journal of Allergy and Clinical Immunology. 2024;**153**(4):988-997.e11. DOI: 10.1016/j.jaci.2023.11.915

[66] Salter BM, Aw M, Sehmi R. The role of type 2 innate lymphoid cells in eosinophilic asthma. Journal of Leukocyte Biology. 2019;**106**:889-901. DOI: 10.1002/JLB.3MR1217-497R

[67] Kato A. Group 2 innate lymphoid cells in airway diseases. Chest. 2019;**156**(1):141-149. DOI: 10.1016/j.chest.2019.04.101

[68] Wallrapp A, Riesenfeld SJ, Burkett PR, et al. The neuropeptide NMU amplifies ILC2-driven allergic lung inflammation. Nature. 2017;**549**(7672):351-356. DOI: 10.1038/nature24029

[69] Mjösberg J, Bernink J, Golebski K, et al. The transcription factor GATA3 is essential for the function of human type 2 innate lymphoid cells. Immunity. 2012;**37**(4):649-659. DOI: 10.1016/j.immuni.2012.08.015

[70] Halim TYF, Steer CA, Mathä L, et al. Group 2 innate lymphoid cells are critical for the initiation of adaptive T helper 2 cell-mediated allergic lung inflammation. Immunity. 2014;**40**(3):425-435. DOI: 10.1016/j.immuni.2014.01.011

[71] Smith SG, Chen R, Kjarsgaard M, et al. Increased numbers of activated group 2 innate lymphoid cells in the airways of patients with severe asthma and persistent airway eosinophilia. The Journal of Allergy and Clinical Immunology. 2016;**137**(1):75-86.e8. DOI: 10.1016/j.jaci.2015.05.037

[72] Shakoory B, Fitzgerald SM, Lee SA, et al. The role of human mast cell-derived cytokines in eosinophil biology. Journal of Interferon and Cytokine Research. 2004;**24**(5):271-281. DOI: 10.1089/107999004323065057

[73] Sakuishi K, Oki S, Araki M. Invariant NKT cells biased for IL-5 production act as crucial regulators of inflammation. Journal of Immunology. 2007;**179**(6):3452-3462. DOI: 10.4049/jimmunol.179.6.3452

[74] Yanagibashi T, Satoh M, Nagai Y, et al. Allergic diseases: From bench to clinic—Contribution of the discovery of interleukin-5. Cytokine. 2017;**98**:59-70. DOI: 10.1016/j.cyto.2016.11.011

[75] Gutierrez-Ramos JC, Lloyd C, Gonzalo JA. Eotaxin: From an eosinophilic chemokine to a major regulator of allergic reactions. Immunology Today. 1999;**20**(11):500-504. DOI: 10.1016/s0167-5699(99)01522-4

[76] Joubert P, Lajoie-Kadoch S, Labonté I, et al. CCR3 expression and function in asthmatic airway smooth muscle cells. Journal of Immunology. 2005;**175**(4):2702-2708. DOI: 10.4049/jimmunol.175.4.2702

[77] Galdiero MR, Varricchi G, Seaf M, et al. Bidirectional mast cell-eosinophil interactions in inflammatory disorders and cancer. Frontiers in Medicine. 2017;**4**:103. DOI: 10.3389/fmed.2017.00103

[78] He K, Hettinga A, Kale SL, et al. Blimp-1 is essential for allergen-induced asthma and Th2 cell development in the lung. The Journal of Experimental Medicine. 2020;**217**:e20190742. DOI: 10.1084/jem.20190742

[79] Petsky HL, Cates CJ, Kew KM, Chang AB. Tailoring asthma treatment on eosinophilic markers (exhaled nitric oxide or sputum eosinophils): A systematic review and meta-analysis. Thorax. 2018;**73**(12):1110-1119. DOI: 10.1136/thoraxjnl-2018-211540

[80] Vermeer PD, Harson R, Einwalter LA, et al. Interleukin-9 induces goblet cell hyperplasia during repair of human airway epithelia. American Journal of Respiratory Cell and Molecular Biology. 2003;**28**(3):286-295. DOI: 10.1165/rcmb.4887

[81] Venegas Garrido C, Mukherjee M, Svenningsen S, Nair P. Eosinophil-mucus interplay in severe asthma: Implications for treatment with biologicals. Allergology International. 2024;**73**(3):351-361. DOI: 10.1016/j.alit.2024.03.001

[82] Zustakova M, Kratochvilova L, Slama P. Apoptosis of eosinophil granulocytes. Biology (Basel). 2020;**9**:457. DOI: 10.3390/biology9120457

[83] Bajbouj K, AbuJabal R, Sahnoon L, et al. IL-5 receptor expression in lung fibroblasts: Potential role in airway remodeling in asthma. Allergy. 2023;**78**:882-885. DOI: 10.1111/all.15627

[84] Maglio A, Vitale C, Pelaia C, et al. Severe asthma remissions induced by biologics targeting IL5/IL5r: Results from a multicenter real-life study. International Journal of Molecular Sciences. 2023;**24**:2455. DOI: 10.3390/ijms24032455

[85] Koranteng J, Chung KF, Michaeloudes C, Bhavsar P. The role of mitochondria in eosinophil function: Implications for severe asthma pathogenesis. Frontiers in Cell and Development Biology. 2024;**12**:1360079. DOI: 10.3389/fcell.2024.1360079

[86] Mauser PJ, Pitman AM, Fernandez X, et al. Effects of an antibody to interleukin-5 in a monkey model of asthma. American Journal of Respiratory and Critical Care Medicine. 1995;**152**(2):467-472. DOI: 10.1164/ajrccm.152.2.7633694

[87] Garlisi CG, Kung TT, Wang P, et al. Effects of chronic anti-interleukin-5 monoclonal antibody treatment in a murine model of pulmonary inflammation. American Journal of Respiratory Cell and Molecular Biology. 1999;**20**(2):248-255. DOI: 10.1165/ajrcmb.20.2.3327

[88] Pavord ID, Bel EH, Bourdin A, et al. From DREAM to REALITI-A and beyond: Mepolizumab for the treatment of eosinophil-driven diseases. Allergy. 2022;**77**(3):778-797. DOI: 10.1111/all.15056

[89] Yancey SW, Keene ON, Albers FC, et al. Biomarkers for severe eosinophilic asthma. The Journal of Allergy and Clinical Immunology. 2017;**140**:1509-1518. DOI: 10.1016/j.jaci.2017.10.005

[90] Pelaia C, Calabrese C, Vatrella A, et al. Benralizumab: From the basic mechanism of action to the potential use in the biological therapy of severe eosinophilic asthma. BioMed Research International. 2018;**2018**:4839230. DOI: 10.1155/2018/4839230

[91] Walsh GM. Reslizumab in the treatment of severe eosinophilic asthma: An update. Immunotherapy. 2018;**10**(8):695-698. DOI: 10.2217/imt-2017-0176

[92] Flood-Page PT, Menzies-Gow AN, Kay AB, Robinson DS. Eosinophil role remains uncertain as anti-interleukin-5 only partially depletes numbers in asthmatic airways. American Journal of Respiratory and Critical Care Medicine. 2003;**167**:199-204. DOI: 10.1164/rccm.200208-789OC

[93] Pelaia C, Vatrella A, Busceti MT, et al. Severe eosinophilic asthma: From the pathogenic role of interleukin-5 to the therapeutic action of mepolizumab. Drug Design, Development and Therapy. 2017;**11**:3137-3144. DOI: 10.2147/DDDT.S150656

[94] Abonia JP, Putnam PE. Mepolizumab in eosinophilic disorders. Expert Review of Clinical Immunology. 2011;7(4):411-417. DOI: 10.1586/eci.11.27

[95] Kusano S, Kukimoto-Niino M, Hino N, et al. Structural basis of interleukin-5 dimer recognition by its α receptor. Protein Science. 2012;**21**(6):850-864. DOI: 10.1002/pro.2072

[96] Mukherjee M, Sehmi R, Nair P. Anti-IL5 therapy for asthma and beyond. World Allergy Organization Journal. 2014;7(1):32. DOI: 10.1186/1939-4551-7-32. eCollection 2014

[97] Leckie MJ, Brinke AT, Khan J, et al. Effects of an interleukin-5 blocking monoclonal antibody on eosinophils, airway hyper-responsiveness, and the late asthmatic response. Lancet. 2000;**356**(9248):2144-2148. DOI: 10.1016/s0140-6736(00)03496-6

[98] Kips JC, O'Connor BJ, Langley SJ, et al. Effect of SCH55700, a humanized anti-human interleukin-5 antibody, in severe persistent asthma: A pilot study. American Journal of Respiratory and Critical Care Medicine. 2003;**167**(12):1655-1659. DOI: 10.1164/rccm.200206-525OC

[99] Haldar P, Brightling CE, Hargadon B, et al. Mepolizumab and exacerbations of refractory eosinophilic asthma. The New England Journal of Medicine. 2009;**360**(10):973-984. DOI: 10.1056/NEJMoa0808991

[100] Pavord ID, Korn S, Howarth P, et al. Mepolizumab for severe eosinophilic asthma (DREAM): A multicentre, double-blind, placebo-controlled trial. Lancet. 2012;**380**(9842):651-659. DOI: 10.1016/S0140-6736(12)60988-X

[101] Ortega HG, Liu MC, Pavord ID, et al. Mepolizumab treatment in patients with severe eosinophilic asthma. The New England Journal of Medicine. 2014;**371**(13):1198-1207. DOI: 10.1056/NEJMoa1403290

[102] Bergantini L, Pianigiani T, d'Alessandro M, et al. The effect of anti-IL5 monoclonal antibodies on regulatory and effector T cells in severe eosinophilic asthma. Biomedicine and Pharmacotherapy. 2023;**166**:115385. DOI: 10.1016/j.biopha.2023.115385

[103] Halwani R, Al-Muhsen S, Al-Jahdali H, Hamid Q. Role of transforming growth factor-β in airway remodeling in asthma. American Journal of Respiratory Cell and Molecular Biology. 2011;**44**(2):127-133. DOI: 10.1165/rcmb.2010-0027TR

[104] Crimi C, Campisi R, Nolasco S, et al. Mepolizumab effectiveness in patients with severe eosinophilic asthma and co-presence of bronchiectasis: A real-world retrospective pilot study. Respiratory Medicine. 2021;**185**:106491. DOI: 10.1016/j.rmed.2021.106491

[105] Deeks ED, Brusselle G. Reslizumab in eosinophilic asthma: A review. Drugs. 2017;**77**(7):777-784. DOI: 10.1007/s40265-017-0740-2

[106] Ibrahim H, O'Sullivan R, Casey D, et al. The effectiveness of reslizumab in severe asthma treatment: A real-world experience. Respiratory Research. 2019;**20**(1):289. DOI: 10.1186/s12931-019-1251-3

[107] Lam J, Hay JW, Salcedo J, Kenyon NJ. A cost-effectiveness analysis of reslizumab in the treatment of poorly controlled eosinophilic asthma. The Journal of Asthma. 2019;**56**(8):872-881. DOI: 10.1080/02770903.2018.1500584

[108] Kavanagh JE, Hearn AP, Dhariwal J, et al. Real-world effectiveness of benralizumab in severe eosinophilic asthma. Chest. 2021;**159**(2):496-506. DOI: 10.1016/j.chest.2020.08.2083

[109] Pham TH, Damera G, Newbold P, Ranade K. Reductions in eosinophil biomarkers by benralizumab in patients with asthma. Respiratory Medicine. 2016;**111**:21-29. DOI: 10.1016/j.rmed.2016.01.003

[110] Marichal T, Mesnil C, Bureau F. Homeostatic eosinophils: Characteristics and functions. Frontiers in Medicine (Lausanne). 2017;**4**:101. DOI: 10.3389/fmed.2017.00101

[111] Van Hulst G, Jorssen J, Jacobs N, et al. Anti-IL5 mepolizumab minimally influences residual blood eosinophils in severe asthma. The European Respiratory Journal. 2022;**59**(3):2100935. DOI: 10.1183/13993003.00935-2021

[112] Mesnil C, Raulier S, Paulissen G, et al. Lung-resident eosinophils represent a distinct regulatory eosinophil subset. The Journal of Clinical Investigation. 2016;**126**(9):3279-3295. DOI: 10.1172/JCI85664

[113] Jackson DJ, Korn S, Mathur SK, et al. Safety of eosinophil-depleting therapy for severe, eosinophilic asthma: Focus on benralizumab. Drug Safety. 2020;**43**(5):409-425. DOI: 10.1007/s40264-020-00926-3

[114] Luo J, Chen W, Liu W, et al. IL-5 antagonism reverses priming and activation of eosinophils in severe eosinophilic asthma. Mucosal Immunology. 2024;**S1933-0219**(24):00024-00022. DOI: 10.1016/j.mucimm.2024.03.005

[115] McCormick SM, Heller NM. Commentary: IL-4 and IL-13 receptors

and signaling. Cytokine. 2015;**75**(1):38-50. DOI: 10.1016/j.cyto.2015.05.023

[116] Wenzel S, Ford L, Pearlman D, et al. Dupilumab in persistent asthma with elevated eosinophil levels. The New England Journal of Medicine. 2013;**368**:2455-2466. DOI: 10.1056/NEJMoa1304048

[117] Xiong XF, Zhu M, Wu HX, et al. Efficacy and safety of dupilumab for the treatment of uncontrolled asthma: A meta-analysis of randomized clinical trials. Respiratory Research. 2019;**20**(1):108. DOI: 10.1186/s12931-019-1065-3

[118] Bacharier LB, Guilbert TW, Katelaris CH, et al. Dupilumab improves lung function parameters in pediatric type 2 asthma: VOYAGE study. The Journal of Allergy and Clinical Immunology. In Practice. 2024;**12**(4):948-959. DOI: 10.1016/j.jaip.2023.12.006

[119] Casale TB, Luskin AT, Busse W, et al. Omalizumab effectiveness by biomarker status in patients with asthma: Evidence from PROSPERO, a prospective real-world study. The Journal of Allergy and Clinical Immunology. In Practice. 2019;**7**(1):156-164.e1. DOI: 10.1016/j.jaip.2018.04.043

[120] Wechsler ME, Munitz A, Ackerman SJ, et al. Eosinophils in health and disease: A state-of-the-art review. Mayo Clinic Proceedings. 2021;**96**(10):2694-2707. DOI: 10.1016/j.mayocp.2021.04.025

[121] Rojo-Tolosa S, González-Gutiérrez MV, Jiménez-Gálvez G, et al. Impact of anti-IL5 therapies on patients with severe uncontrolled asthma and possible predictive biomarkers of response: A real-life study. International Journal of Molecular Sciences. 2023;**24**:2011. DOI: 10.3390/ijms24032011

[122] Kimura Y, Suzukawa M, Inoue N, et al. Differences in asthma-related outcomes by anti-IL-5 biologics, omalizumab, and dupilumab based on blood eosinophil counts. Asian Pacific Journal of Allergy and Immunology. 2024. DOI: 10.12932/AP-290623-1645 [Epub ahead of print]

[123] Pfeffer PE, Ali N, Murray R, et al. Comparative effectiveness of anti-IL5 and anti-IgE biologic classes in patients with severe asthma eligible for both. Allergy. 2023;**78**:1934-1948. DOI: 10.1111/all.15711

[124] Charles D, Shanley J, Temple SN, et al. Real-world efficacy of treatment with benralizumab, dupilumab, mepolizumab and reslizumab for severe asthma: A systematic review and meta-analysis. Clinical and Experimental Allergy. 2022;**52**:616-627. DOI: 10.1111/cea.14112

[125] Bourdin A, Brusselle G, Couillard S, et al. Phenotyping of severe asthma in the era of broad-acting anti-asthma biologics. The Journal of Allergy and Clinical Immunology. In Practice. 2024;**12**(4):809-823. DOI: 10.1016/j.jaip.2024.01.023

[126] Oppenheimer J, Hoyte FCL, Phipatanakul W, et al. Allergic and eosinophilic asthma in the era of biomarkers and biologics: Similarities, differences and misconceptions. Annals of Allergy, Asthma and Immunology. 2022;**129**(2):169-180. DOI: 10.1016/j.anai.2022.02.021

[127] Nyenhuis SM, Krishnan JA, Berry A, et al. Race is associated with differences in airway inflammation in patients with asthma. The Journal of Allergy and Clinical Immunology. 2017;**140**(1):257-265.e11. DOI: 10.1016/j.jaci.2016.10.024

Chapter 4

A Note on the Biological Functions and Activities of Eosinophils

Odewusi Odeyinka Olufunsho and Omon Emmanuel Akokhamen

Abstract

Eosinophils are a class of white blood cells named after the ability of their cytoplasmic granules to take up the acidic part of the Romanowsky group of stains. Eosinophils are primarily produced in the bone marrow during the process of leucopoiesis—the production of white blood cells. After maturation, the white blood cell subsets with bilobed nuclei, and pinkish eosinophilic cytoplasmic granules are released into the circulation. From here, they migrate to various parts of the body. The drumstick appendage possessed by eosinophil of females is the only but striking distinguishing feature between eosinophils from both genders. Eosinophils produce various cytokines that activate other blood cells in the inflammatory response, wound healing, and hemopoiesis. The presence of eosinophils in some tissues where they do not normally reside as well as their increase in population in tissues where they can be found signify parasitic infection. This may not confirm a diagnosis but will nonetheless be a pointer toward the direction of confirming or ruling out a diagnosis. Their presence or population can also be used in assessing the severity as well as monitoring the progress of the parasitic infection.

Keywords: eosinophils, inflammation, infection, immunity, white blood cells

1. Introduction

Eosinophils are a subset of white blood cells crucial for various vertebrate biological functions, particularly in defending against parasitic infections. They are involved in regulating allergy and asthma, along with mast cells and basophils. Eosinophils are granulocytes that proliferate during hematopoiesis in the bone marrow and then go into circulation. Once in the bloodstream, they undergo terminal differentiation and cease to proliferate [1]. Eosinophils, which have bilobed nuclei and measure between 12 and 17 micrometers in size, normally comprise 1–3% of white blood cells in healthy persons. While eosinophils are released into the bloodstream, their primary locations are in the thymus, lower gastrointestinal tract, ovaries, uterus, spleen, and lymph nodes. They are not normally found in the lungs, skin, esophagus, or some other internal organs; the presence of eosinophils in these organs is typically indicative of disease. Eosinophils can survive in tissue for an extra 8–12 days without external stimulation [2].

Eosinophils are multifunctional white blood cells that are involved in a number of inflammatory processes, such as tissue damage, tumor immunity, bacterial and viral infections, and allergy disorders. Eosinophils are drawn from the circulation and

 IntechOpen

brought to areas of inflammation in response to numerous stimuli, where they employ several mechanisms to regulate immune responses [3]. Interleukin (IL)-2, IL-4, IL-5, IL-10, IL-12, IL-13, IL-16, IL-18, and transforming growth factor (TGF)-a/b are examples of proinflammatory cytokines that can be secreted by activated eosinophils via the engagement of complement, immunoglobulin, and cytokine receptors. Other chemokines that can be secreted include CCL5/RANTES and CCL11/eotaxin-1 and lipid mediators like platelet-activating factor (PAF) and leukotriene (LT)C4. The increase of adhesion systems, modification of cellular trafficking and activation, control of vascular permeability, secretion of mucus, and constriction of smooth muscle are among the proinflammatory effects of these molecules. By serving as antigen-presenting cells, eosinophils can also trigger immunological responses specific to particular antigens. Furthermore, they have the ability to release lipid mediators and toxic granule proteins, which can lead to tissue injury and malfunction [4].

Granule proteins and chemical mediators produced by eosinophils may be involved in tissue damage, repair, remodeling, and disease persistence in conditions like asthma, chronic rhinosinusitis with nasal polyps (CRSwNP), eosinophilic gastrointestinal (GI) disorders, and systemic hypereosinophilic diseases like eosinophilic granulomatosis with polyangiitis (EGPA) and hypereosinophilic syndrome (HES). One important cytokine that plays a role in eosinophil recruitment, activation, maturation, and proliferation is interleukin (IL)-5. IL-4 and IL-13 are two additional cytokines linked to tissue eosinophil recruitment and type 2 (T2) immune responses typified by eosinophilia. These cytokines are therefore targets for therapeutic approaches [5].

1.1 Physiology and biology of eosinophil

Various cytotoxic granule cationic proteins, such as eosinophil cationic protein (ECP), eosinophil peroxidase (EPO), eosinophil-derived neurotoxin (EDN), and major basic protein (MBP), are secreted by eosinophils and can cause tissue damage and malfunction [6]. MBP-1 (and MBP2) make up the crystalloid core of eosinophil granules, while ECP, EDN, and EPO make up the matrix. Heart, brain, and bronchial epithelium are among the tissues that are hazardous to MBP, EPO, and ECP. Both ribonucleases, ECP and EDN, have been demonstrated to exhibit antiviral action. ECP creates voltage-insensitive, ion-selective harmful gaps in target cell membranes, which may allow other cytotoxic compounds to enter the cell [7]. In addition, ECP has several other noncytotoxic effects, such as promoting the creation of glycosaminoglycan by human fibroblasts and secreting mucus from the airways, inducing mast cell degranulation, and suppressing T cell proliferative responses and immunoglobulin synthesis by B cells. By deregulating the function of vagal muscarinic M2 and M3 receptors and causing mast cell and basophil degranulation, MBP directly modifies the responses of smooth muscle contraction. Recent research has linked MBP to the control of peripheral nerve plasticity. EPO, which makes up approximately 25% of the total protein mass of certain granules, catalyzes the formation of highly reactive oxygen species (hypohalous acids) and reactive nitrogen metabolites (perioxynitrate) by oxidizing pseudohalides [thyiocyanate (SCN−)], halides [chloride (Cl−), bromide (Br−), iodide (I−)], and nitric oxide (nitrite). These substances oxidize protein nucleophilic targets, causing oxidative stress, necrosis, and apoptosis that lead to cell death [8].

Eosinophils primarily secrete their granule protein by controlled degranulation and exocytosis. Piecemeal degranulation is the process by which eosinophils release particular granule components one at a time. When IFN-γ activates human eosinophils, for instance, granule-derived RANTES are mobilized to the cell periphery without causing the release of cationic proteins. A docking complex consisting of soluble N-ethylmaleimide-sensitive factor attachment protein (SNAREs) on the vesicle (v-SNAREs) and target membrane (t-SNAREs) mediates regulated exocytosis. The presence of arginine [R] or glutamine [Q], two conserved amino acids, divides SNAREs into two groups. The Q-SNAREs SNAP-23 and syntaxin-4, which are mostly found in the plasma membrane, and the R-SNARE VAMP (vesicle-associated membrane protein)-2, which is found in cytoplasmic secretory vesicles, are expressed by human eosinophils. The hypothesis suggests that when eosinophils are activated via receptors, cytoplasmic vesicles are quickly mobilized to the plasma membrane. This results in the creation of a SNARE complex (VAMP2/SNAP-23/syntaxin-4) and the subsequent release of mediators [9].

1.2 Development of eosinophil

In the bone marrow, pluripotent stem cells give rise to eosinophils after differentiating into a hybrid precursor that shares characteristics with basophils and eosinophils and subsequently into a distinct eosinophil lineage. At least three types of transcription factors, including GATA-1 (a zinc family finger member), PU.1 (a member of the erythroblast transformation specific (ETS) family), and C/EBP members (CCAAT/enhancer-binding protein family), interact to determine the specification of the eosinophil lineage. Despite being expressed throughout a range of hematologic lineages, these transcription factors operate differently in eosinophils. Specifically, PU.1 expression levels indicate diverse cell lineage fates; low expression indicates lymphocytic differentiation, while high expression indicates myeloid differentiation. GATA-1 and PU.1 have a negative functional relationship in the majority of cell types, but they work together to control the transcription of eosinophil granule protein and eosinophil lineage specification [10].

The regulation of eosinophil growth is mostly dependent on three cytokines: IL-3, IL-5, and GM-CSF. Following the instructional signals provided by the transcription factors GATA-1, PU.1, and C/EBPs, these eosinophilopoietins most likely offer permissive proliferation and differentiation signals. On chromosome 5q31, these cytokines are encoded by closely related genes. They attach themselves to receptors that have distinct alpha chains and a shared beta chain [11]. Out of the three cytokines, IL-5 is the one that is most specific to the eosinophil lineage and is in charge of eosinophils' selective differentiation. Additionally, eosinophils in the bone marrow are stimulated by IL-5 to discharge into the peripheral circulation. Mice genetic manipulation provides the greatest example of the crucial function IL-5 plays in eosinophil production. When the IL-5 gene is deleted, eosinophil counts in the blood and lungs following an allergen challenge are significantly reduced. This results in severe eosinophilia in transgenic mice that overproduce IL-5 [1]. When a person has eosinophilia, they overproduce one or more of these three cytokines, and diseases that cause selective eosinophilia frequently also cause overproduction of IL-5. Clinical experiments using humanized anti-IL-5 antibody have shown the crucial function that IL-5 plays in regulating human eosinophils; this currently unapproved treatment significantly reduces eosinophil levels in the blood and to a lesser extent in the inflamed lung [2].

1.3 Functions of eosinophils

1.3.1 Homeostatic function

Because eosinophils and parasite infections have been linked in early clinical studies, researchers have postulated that eosinophils are end-stage effector cells that are traditionally implicated in host defense. However, eosinophils have been linked to a number of biological processes in recent times, such as the development of the postpubertal mammary gland, the cycle of estrus, organ transplantation, viral infection, allergic inflammatory reactions, and neoplasia [11].

1.3.2 Eosinophils and reproduction

In the female reproductive tract, eosinophils are a common cell population that reaches their peak quantity during estrus. Eosinophils are primarily found in the endometrial-myometrial junction and in the endometrial stroma, which is next to the luminal and glandular epithelium. The uterine eosinophil population is reduced in IL5-deficient mice, but there is still a residual population of eosinophils, and their location in the subepithelial stroma is similar to that of wild-type mice. This suggests that IL-5-independent mechanisms control the recruitment of eosinophils into the uterus according to tissue specificity [3]. To support this idea, eosinophil infiltration into the uterus is correlated with the upregulation of eotaxin-1, RANTES, and MIP-1α, three eosinophil-active chemokines, in response to ovarian steroid hormones. In fact, eotaxin-1-deficient animals lack uterine eosinophils and exhibit a two-week delay in the onset of estrus and the first age of parturition, indicating that eosinophils can play a role in preparing the mature uterus for pregnancy. Moreover, in the aftermath of copulation, eosinophils penetrate the endometrium, and scientists have speculated that this cell might play a part in blastocyst implantation and infection defense, albeit this has not been demonstrated [4].

The development of the mammary glands after birth has also been linked to eosinophils. The postnatal growing mammary gland is home to eosinophils, which are primarily found at the terminal end buds' heads. Between 0 and 4 weeks of age, eotaxin-1 mRNA expression is modest; by the time the child is 5 weeks old, the mammary gland has experienced a large increase in this gene. Notably, at this point, eosinophil infiltration into the head of the terminal end bud corresponds with increased expression of eotaxin-1. Terminal end bud development and branching complexity of the ductal tree are reduced when eosinophils from the postnatal mammary gland are depleted through deletion of the eotaxin-1 gene. Eosinophil-derived TGF-β is probably secreted locally by eosinophils to control mammary gland ductal expansion [12].

1.3.3 Thymic eosinophils

During the neonatal stage, eosinophils move into the thymus, localize in the corticomedullary area, and multiply to their highest concentration by 2 weeks of age. Fascinatingly, their absolute concentrations are roughly equal to those of thymic dendritic cells. The medullary area is where eosinophils localize [7]. Eosinophils mostly settle in the thymus's corticomedullary area, where they attain basal levels by 28 days of life. Consequently, the start of thymic involution is correlated with a rise in thymic eosinophil levels around 16 weeks of age. Interestingly, at this stage, eosinophils localize to the medullary area. Thymic eosinophils exhibit the costimulatory markers CD86 (B7.2) and CD30L (CD153), as well as high amounts of MHC class II and moderate levels of MHC class I molecules. Thymic eosinophil cytokine production analysis shows that eosinophils express mRNA for Th2-cytokines, IL-4 and IL-13, and proinflammatory cytokines, TNF-α, TGF-β, IL1α, and IL-6. Notably, eotaxin-1, which is constitutively expressed in the thymus, regulates the recruitment of eosinophils into the thymus. Eosinophils are thought to be linked to MHC class I-restricted thymocyte deletion. The idea that double-positive thymocytes are negatively selected is supported by the biphasic recruitment of eosinophils and their anatomical location inside distinct compartments of the thymus [5].

1.4 Eosinophils and immune regulation

Through the production of a variety of mostly preformed cytokines and lipid mediators, researchers have demonstrated in recent years that eosinophils are capable of carrying out a wide range of immunological tasks, including antigen presentation and escalation of inflammatory reactions.

1.4.1 Antigen presentation

Many antigens from bacteria, viruses, and parasites can be processed and presented by eosinophils. Furthermore, eosinophils treated with granulocyte-macrophage colony-stimulating factor (GM-CSF) stimulate T cell proliferation in response to staphylococcal superantigen (*Staphylococcus enterotoxins* A, B, and E) stimulation. Additionally, the proliferation of T cells specific to rhinovirus-16 and the release of IFN-γ are stimulated by eosinophils cultured with human rhinovirus-16. Moreover, eosinophils can function well. Numerous cytokines (IL-2, IL-4, IL-6, IL-10, and IL-12) secreted by eosinophils have the ability to stimulate T cell proliferation, activation, and Th1/Th2 polarization. The capacity of murine eosinophils to generate IL-4 has garnered interest recently. It is interesting to note that eosinophils appear to produce less IL-4 protein than basophils and T cells, despite the fact that the IL4 gene locus is transcriptionally active. Moreover, CD4+ T cells secrete IL-4, IL-5, and IL-13 in response to murine eosinophils. By synthesizing indoleamine 2,3-dioxygenase (IDO), an enzyme involved in the oxidative metabolism of tryptophan and the conversion of tryptophan to kynurenines (KYN), eosinophils can also control T cell polarization. By encouraging Th1 cell death, KYN controls the imbalance between Th1 and Th2. Costimulation is necessary for the eosinophil-mediated T cell proliferative and cytokine production responses. In fact, neutralizing antibodies that block CD80, CD86, and CTLA-4 prevent T cells from proliferating and secreting cytokines when eosinophils are present [13].

1.4.2 Mast cell regulation

The ability of eosinophils to control mast cell function has been shown in a large body of research. Notably, MBP can activate mast cells generated from human umbilical cord blood, causing the release of histamine, PGD-2, GM-CSF, TNF-α, and IL-8. In addition to exocytosis, MBP-stimulated mast cell activation triggers the synthesis of cytokines and eicosanoid, both of which are important reactions that accompany Fc/RI-dependent mast cell activation. Rat peritoneal mast cells exhibit concentration-dependent histamine release when cultured with natural MBP, EPO, and ECP (but not EDN) [14]. It has been demonstrated that MBP activates mast cells through a mechanism resembling that of other polybasic substances such substance P, compound 48/80, and bradykinin. Highly pure lung mast cells cocultured with human lung fibroblasts are vulnerable to IgE-independent activation by MBP, whereas freshly separated human lung mast cells are resistant to IgE-independent activation. It is interesting to note that eosinophil-derived stem cell factor, a vital mast cell growth factor, is produced more readily when eosinophils are activated with the mast cell protease chymase. Additionally, nerve growth factor (NGF), a cytokine important in immunological control as well as sympathetic neuron survival and function, is produced by eosinophils. NGF, for instance, encourages mast cell activation and survival. Eosinophils produce NGF, which operates in an autocrine manner by triggering the release of EPO. Histamine is released by rat peritoneal muscles when EPO is applied, indicating that mast cell–eosinophil interactions may involve eosinophil-derived NGF. Therefore, there is bidirectional communication between mast cells and eosinophils [15].

1.5 Clinical significance

Eosinophilia, defined as having more than 500 eosinophils/microlitre of blood, is commonly observed in patients with intestinal parasite infestations, autoimmune and collagen vascular diseases (like rheumatoid arthritis) and Systemic lupus erythematosus; malignant diseases like eosinophilic leukemia, clonal hypereosinophilia, and Hodgkin lymphoma; lymphocyte-variant hypereosinophilia; extensive skin conditions (like exfoliative dermatitis); Addison's disease and other conditions resulting in low corticosteroid production (corticosteroids suppress blood eosinophil levels); reflux esophagitis (where eosinophils are found in the squamous epithelium of the esophagus) and eosinophilic esophagitis; and with the use of certain medications like penicillin. However, an allergy disease like asthma may be the most frequent cause of eosinophilia [16].

The quantity of accumulating eosinophils correlates with the severity of an asthmatic reaction, suggesting that eosinophils are significant in asthma. There is evidence linking elevated interleukin-5 levels to eosinophilia in mouse models. In addition, higher levels of interleukin-5 have been reported to result in higher amounts of eosinophils in mucosal bronchial biopsies performed on individuals with disorders like asthma. These elevated eosinophil infiltration levels result in an inflammatory response. The end result of this is breathing difficulties and remodeling of the airways. In the lungs of asthmatic individuals, eosinophils can also degrade lung tissue. The lungs' degranulation sites and the sputum produced by asthmatics include high amounts of eosinophil major basic protein and eosinophil-derived neurotoxic, which are almost cytotoxic [17].

1.6 Role of eosinophils in disease

1.6.1 Infections

The primary role of eosinophils in aiding the host against parasitic helminths has been identified as their positive function. The ability of eosinophils to mediate antibody- (or complement-) dependent cellular toxicity against helminths in vitro, the observation that eosinophil levels increase during helminthic infections, and the fact that eosinophils aggregate and degranulate in the local vicinity of damaged parasites in vivo, and the outcomes in experimental parasite-infected mice that have had their eosinophils depleted by IL-5 neutralization and/or gene targeting are the various lines of evidence that support this theory [18]. It is important to interpret these in vivo findings cautiously because IL-5 neutralization may affect human basophils, murine B cells, and probably human pulmonary smooth muscle cells, among other cells that contain the IL-5 receptor. Recent methods have revealed a role for eosinophils in the encystment of larvae in Trichinella spiralis and in controlling the Brugiamalayi microfilariae, respectively. These methods include the investigation of CCR3- and eotaxin-1-deficient mice. Maybe examination of freshly created eosinophil-deficient mice after experimental parasite infection will offer further strong proof that eosinophils are involved in host defense against parasites. It appears probable that eosinophils contribute to the protective immunity against some helminths, despite the controversy reported in various research [14, 18].

There is growing evidence that eosinophils may also operate as defenses against other diseases, particularly against RNA viruses like respiratory syncytial virus (RSV) and the associated pneumonia virus of mice (PVM), which is a natural rodent pathogen. Significantly, several ribonucleases that break down viruses containing single-stranded RNA are found in eosinophil granule proteins. These ribonucleases include human ECP and EDN as well as at least 11 orthologs of eosinophil-associated ribonuclease (EAR) in mice. When compared to other primates, ECP and EDN are really the most divergent coding sequences in the entire human genome. They have maintained ribonuclease activity across species in spite of their divergence, which clearly suggests that there is evolutionary pressure to maintain this essential enzyme activity [9].

1.6.2 Asthma

Bronchoalveolar lavage fluid from asthmatic patients has been discovered to have elevated quantities of eosinophil granule proteins (e.g., MBP). Interestingly, these concentrations are high enough to cause cytotoxicity of a range of host tissue, including respiratory epithelial cells *in vitro*. MBP-induced basophil and mast cell direct degranulation are assumed to play a role in the etiology of disease [19]. Apart from its cytotoxic effects, MBP also causes malfunction of vagal muscarinic M2 receptors, which increases smooth muscle responsiveness directly. This is likely to play a role in the development of airway hyperreactivity (AHR), a hallmark feature of asthma. Furthermore, eosinophils produce a significant number of cysteinyl leukotrienes. Notably, the proteins found in eosinophil granules include all the metabolic components needed to produce cysteinyl leukotrienes. These mediators are strong smooth muscle constrictors that cause an increase in mucus secretion and vascular permeability. Cysteinyl leukotriene inhibitors are, in fact, useful therapeutic tools for the management of allergic respiratory disease [10].

1.6.3 Gastrointestinal disorders

Many conditions, including drug reactions, helminth infections, hypereosinophilic syndromes, eosinophilic gastroenteritis, allergic colitis, inflammatory bowel disease, and gastroesophageal reflux disease, are associated with an accumulation of eosinophils in the gastrointestinal tract [8]. Eosinophilic esophagitis (EE), eosinophilic gastritis, and eosinophilic gastroenteritis are among the conditions that make up a subset of these illnesses known as primary eosinophil-associated gastrointestinal disorders (EGID). These are hypersensitivity conditions that fall between anaphylaxis and celiac disease. Peripheral blood eosinophilia is not always associated with EGID, highlighting the importance of gastrointestinal-specific processes controlling eosinophil counts [6].

1.7 Anti-eosinophil therapeutics

Several medications prevent the formation of eosinophils or compounds produced from them. These consist of leukotriene production or receptor antagonists, glucocorticoids, myelosuppressive medications, tyrosine kinase inhibitors, humanized anti-IL-5 antibodies, and IFN-α. The ideal treatment plan is frequently determined by the etiology of the underlying illness. The best medications for lowering eosinophilia in the majority of other people are glucocorticoids. They inhibit the transcription of several genes that code for inflammatory mediators, including GM-CSF, IL-3, IL-4, and IL-5, as well as a variety of chemokines, such as eotaxins. It has been demonstrated that mRNA instability is the primary mechanism by which glucocorticoids affect eosinophil-active cytokines, hence shortening the half-life of cytokines like eotaxins. Furthermore, cytokine-dependent survival of eosinophils is inhibited by glucocorticoids. Treatment with systemic or topical (intranasal or inhaled) glucocorticoids usually results in a quick decrease in eosinophils; however, some patients develop resistance to the drug and continue to have eosinophilia even at high dosages. Reduced glucocorticoid receptor levels and changes in transcription factor activator protein (AP)-1 appear to be at least partially responsible for the uncertain mechanism of glucocorticoid resistance [20].

Patients who are resistant to corticosteroids may need to consider alternative forms of treatment, such as intracellular retinoid (IFN-α) or myelosuppressive medications like vincristine and hydroxyurea. The fact that IFN-α prevents eosinophil degranulation and effector action makes it particularly useful. It is noteworthy that IFN-α therapy frequently induces remission in patients with myeloproliferative forms of hypereosinophilic syndrome. Another reason cyclophilins, such as cyclosporine A, have been employed is because they prevent the transcription of many cytokines that activate eosinophils, like GM-CSF and IL-5. Eosinophil survival has been demonstrated to be shortened by lidocaine, a noncytotoxic drug whose effects are similar to those of glucocorticoids. Nebulized lidocaine is, in fact, safe and helpful for individuals with asthma, according to early clinical research [16].

Recently licensed leukotriene antagonists and inhibitors are among the medications that obstruct eosinophil chemotactic signals. 5. Lipoxygenase inhibition (e.g., zileuton) prevents the production of the eosinophil chemoattractant LTB4 and the cysteinyl leukotrienes by blocking the rate-limiting step in leukotriene synthesis. Cysteinyl leukotriene receptor antagonists prevent leukocyte-derived leukotrienes from mediating muscle contraction and enhanced vascular permeability. A number of third-generation antihistamines directly inhibit eosinophils in vitro and prevent them from vacuolizing and accumulating after being challenged with allergens. Nedocromil and cromoglycate prevent eosinophil effector functions such as antibody-dependent cellular cytotoxicity [15].

2. Conclusion

For a long time, eosinophils were thought to be end-stage cells that helped shield the host from parasites. Nevertheless, a multitude of lines of evidence have now altered this viewpoint, demonstrating that eosinophils are pleiotropic multifunctional leukocytes engaged in the initiation and spread of many inflammatory responses in addition to modulating adaptive immunity through direct T-cell activation. Eosinophils are expected to have a physiological role as typical components of the mucosal immune system, especially in the gastrointestinal tract. As an early and potentially crucial source of cytokines (like IL-4), eosinophils have been linked to innate immunity. They have also been linked to developmental events including the development of the mammary gland. T cells now regulate eosinophils by an integrated process that includes Th2 cell-derived IL-13 regulating eotaxin synthesis and Th2 cell-derived IL-5 regulating eosinophil growth in the bone marrow and blood. These results suggest that the medical treatment of eosinophilic patients will probably change as a result of targeted therapy against important eosinophil regulators (e.g., humanized anti-IL-5 and CCR3 antagonists).

Author details

Odewusi Odeyinka Olufunsho* and Omon Emmanuel Akokhamen
Department of Medical Laboratory Science, College of Medicine and Health Sciences, Afe Babalola University, Ado Ekiti, Ekiti State, Nigeria

*Address all correspondence to: yinksdaprof@gmail.com

References

[1] Uhm TG, Kim BS, Chung IY. Eosinophil development, regulation of eosinophil-specific genes, and role of eosinophils in the pathogenesis of asthma. Allergy, Asthma & Immunology Research. 2021;**4**(2):68-79

[2] Abdala-Valencia H, Coden ME, Chiarella SE. Shaping eosinophil identity in the tissue contextsof development, homeostasis, and disease. Journal of Leukocyte Biology. 2018;**104**(1):95-108

[3] McBrien CN, Menzies-Gow A. The biology of eosinophils and their role in asthma. Frontiers in Medicine (Lausanne). 2017;**4**:93

[4] Klion A. Recent advances in understanding eosinophil biology. F1000Res. 2019;**8**:1084

[5] Acharya KR, Ackerman SJ. Eosinophil granule proteins: Form and function. The Journal of Biological Chemistry. 2018;**289**(25):17406-17415

[6] Flores-TorresAS,Salinas-CarmonaMC, Salinas E, RosasTaraco AG. Eosinophils and respiratory viruses. Viral Immunology. 2019;**32**(5):198-207

[7] Loktionov A. Eosinophils in the gastrointestinal tract and their role in the pathogenesis of major colorectal disorders. World Journal of Gastroenterology. 2019;**25**(27):3503-3526

[8] Brigger D, Riether C, van Brummelen R. Eosinophils regulate adipose tissue inflammation and sustain physical and immunological fitness in old age. Nature Metabolism. 2020;**2**(8):688-702

[9] Hartl S, Breyer MK, Burghuber OC. Blood eosinophil count in the general population: Typical values and potential confounders. The European Respiratory Journal. 2020;**55**(5):1901874

[10] Grisaru-Tal S, Itan M, Klion AD, Munitz A. A new dawn for eosinophils in the tumour microenvironment. Nature Reviews. Cancer. 2020;**20**(10):594-607

[11] Pavord ID. Blood eosinophil-directed management of airway disease. The past, present, and future. American Journal of Respiratory and Critical Care Medicine. 2020;**202**(5):637-639

[12] Gouon-Evans V, Rothenberg ME, Pollard JW. Postnatal mammary gland development requires macrophages and eosinophils. Development. 2020;**127**:2269-2282

[13] Bandeira-Melo C, Bozza PT, Weller PF. The cellular biology of eosinophil eicosanoid formation and function. Journal of Allergy and Clinical Immunology. 2002;**109**:393-400

[14] Rothenberg ME, Pomerantz JL, Owen WF, Avraham S, Soberman RJ. Characterization of a human eosinophil proteoglycan, and augmentation of its biosynthesis and size by interleukin 3, interleukin 5, and granulocyte/macrophage colony stimulating factor. The Journal of Biological Chemistry. 2018;**263**:13901-13908

[15] MacKenzie JR, Mattes J, Dent LA, Foster PS. Eosinophils promote allergic disease of the lung by regulating CD4+ Th2 lymphocyte function. Journal of Immunology. 2019;**167**:3146-3155

[16] Butterworth AE. The eosinophil and its role in immunity to helminth infection. Current Topics in Microbiology and Immunology. 2019;**77**:127-168

[17] Logan MR, Lacy P, Bablitz B, Moqbel R. Expression of eosinophil target SNAREs as potential cognate receptors for vesicle-associated membrane protein-2 in exocytosis. The Journal of Allergy and Clinical Immunology. 2020;**109**:299-306

[18] Rosenberg HF, Domachowske JB. Eosinophils, eosinophil ribonucleases, and their role in host defense against respiratory virus pathogens. Journal of Leukocyte Biology. 2021;**70**:691-698

[19] Drake MG, Lebold KM, Roth-Carter QR. Eosinophil and airway nerve interactions in asthma. Journal of Leukocyte Biology. 2018;**104**(1):61-67

[20] Weller PF, Spencer LA. Functions of tissue-resident eosinophils. Nature Reviews. Immunology. 2017;**17**(12):746-760

Chapter 5

Eosinophils in Pathology

Rosario Medellin-Vallejo and Barbara Saenz-Ibarra

Abstract

This chapter explores the diverse roles of eosinophils across different tissues and organs, beyond their traditional association with allergies and parasitic infections. From the skin to the cardiovascular system, eosinophils contribute significantly to various physiological and pathological processes. In skin conditions like atopic dermatitis and drug-induced hypersensitivity reactions, eosinophils aggravate itching and inflammation. They also play a role in gastrointestinal diseases like eosinophilic esophagitis and eosinophilic gastritis, where they contribute to tissue damage and inflammation. In the respiratory system, eosinophils are implicated in asthma, eosinophilic pneumonia, and allergic bronchopulmonary aspergillosis, exacerbating airway inflammation and bronchial damage. Additionally, eosinophils are involved in cardiovascular disorders such as eosinophilic myocarditis and hypereosinophilic syndrome, contributing to cardiac inflammation and fibrosis. Understanding the multifaceted roles of eosinophils in different organs is crucial for elucidating disease mechanisms and developing targeted therapies.

Keywords: eosinophil, eosinophilia, eosinophilic, allergic, atopic, asthma, hypersensitivity, urticaria

1. Introduction

Eosinophils are part of the white blood cells responsible for supporting the immune system. Once recognized primarily for their role in allergies and parasitic infections, eosinophils are now understood to play diverse roles in different tissues and organs throughout the human body. From the respiratory system to the gastrointestinal tract, and from the skin to the cardiovascular system, eosinophils contribute significantly to various physiological and pathological processes. This chapter explores the multifaceted roles of eosinophils in different tissues and organs by discussing the most common eosinophilic diseases, offering a comprehensive overview of their clinical significance.

2. Eosinophils on skin

Eosinophilic infiltration is a common finding in various skin conditions, also known as eosinophilic dermatoses, encompassing a wide range of dermatological disorders. However, diagnosing eosinophilic dermatoses can be challenging due to the lack of specific clinical signs, which can occur with or without blood eosinophilia.

Many eosinophilic dermatoses are accompanied by intense itching, such as in atopic dermatitis, prurigo nodularis, bullous pemphigoid and scabies.

Eosinophils are known to aggravate itching by stimulating nerve cells and releasing various substances like granule proteins (eosinophil cationic protein, eosinophil-derived neurotoxin), as well as mediators and cytokines such as substance P, vasoactive intestinal peptide, IL-4, IL-13, and IL-31 [1].

Eosinophilic dermatoses can present with a variety of clinical patterns, each characterized by distinct features and manifestations, in seven distinctive patterns: eczematous pattern, papular rashes, urticarial rashes, blisters and pustules, nodular lesions, vasculitis, and fibrosis. Typically, a combination of clinical manifestations, skin biopsy, and histological analysis is necessary for accurate diagnosis. Hereby are described these main clinical patterns and the most common entities related to them.

2.1 Eczematous pattern

The eczematous pattern refers to dermatoses characterized by pruritic eczema-like skin lesions. Histologic findings include epidermal spongiosis (accumulation of fluid between epidermal cells, leading to intracellular edema), acanthosis (thickening of the epidermis), and dermal eosinophilic infiltrate.

2.1.1 Atopic dermatitis

Atopic Dermatitis (AD) is a common chronic inflammatory skin disease characterized by pruritic eczematous lesions. The prevalence of AD varies across different populations and age groups; it can range between 11.4 and 16.9% during the first 6 years of age [2], while the percentage of adults ever diagnosed with AD by a physician was 4.9% in the USA, 3.5% in Canada, 4.4% in the EU, and 2.1% in Japan [1]. It typically affects the face, neck, and extensor sites of the extremities in infants. The development of this condition relies on a genetic predisposition that leads to both skin barrier dysfunction and the prevalence of type 2 inflammation, influenced by environmental factors [3]. The disease course of AD can vary, with some patients experiencing persistent symptoms into adulthood. In adults, it presents as chronically inflamed lesions with lichenification of the flexural folds.

2.2 Macular and papular rash

The macular and papular rash pattern is characterized by the presence of flat, discolored spots (macules) and small, raised bumps (papules) on the skin. Skin biopsies of these lesions reveal a significant infiltration of eosinophils in the dermis, while skin lesions in drug-induced hypersensitivity reactions with papule formation often reveal hydropic degeneration of keratinocytes, necrosis of keratinocytes, and infiltration of lymphocytes and eosinophils into the dermis and epidermis [4].

2.2.1 Delayed-type drug hypersensitivity reactions

Including macular and papular rashes, Delayed-type Drug Hypersensitivity Reactions (DDHR) are considered to be mainly type IV hypersensitivity reactions mediated by T cells, triggered by medications. CD4+ and CD8+ T cells express perforin and granzyme B, which are key cytotoxic molecules involved in inducing apoptosis in target cells such as activated keratinocytes [4]. Eosinophils are commonly found in the blood and, in varying proportions, in lesional skin. The spectrum of DDHR includes maculopapular exanthema, bullous exanthema, toxic epidermal necrolysis, and the drug hypersensitivity syndrome with varying degrees of eosinophilic infiltrate on the skin.

2.2.2 Drug rash with eosinophilia and systemic symptoms (DRESS)

Drug Rash with Eosinophilia and Systemic Symptoms (DRESS) syndrome is a severe drug reaction characterized by a widespread maculopapular rash, fever, and eosinophilia. Eosinophils play a key role in the pathogenesis of DRESS, with interleukin-5 (IL-5) considered a main driver of eosinophil expansion and activation in this syndrome. It is a delayed hypersensitivity reaction, often triggered by medications, particularly antiepileptic drugs, sulfonamides, and allopurinol, with incidence estimates ranging from 1 in 1000 to 10,000 drug exposures [5]. Even though mortality rates associated with DRESS syndrome are relatively low (5–10%), with full recovery achieved in the majority of cases, it requires prompt recognition and management to avoid multiorgan failure and unpredictable outcomes [1].

2.3 Urticarial pattern

The urticarial pattern in dermatoses is characterized by the development of wheals (hives) on the skin, which are typically raised, pruritic, and erythematous. It is often triggered by allergic reactions to food, medications, or other substances. It is mediated by the release of histamine and other inflammatory mediations, leading to vasodilation and increased vascular permeability.

2.3.1 Urticaria

Urticaria is a skin condition characterized by the sudden appearance of raised, red, and itchy welts on the skin surface. By expressing tissue factor [6], Vascular Endothelial Growth Factor (VEGF), and producing leukotrienes [7], eosinophils have the potential to increase vascular permeability, resulting in dermal edema and the formation of wheals. Histologically, urticaria is characterized by a discrete mixed inflammation in the dermis, which may include eosinophils and dermal edema.

2.4 Blisters and pustules

The blisters and pustules pattern is characterized by the presence of fluid-filled lesions, which can manifest as blisters or pustules; they can vary in size and may be localized or widespread on the skin. Blisters in autoimmune conditions like bullous pemphigoid and pemphigus result from autoantibodies targeting components of the skin's adhesion structures, leading to separation of the epidermis from the dermis.

2.4.1 Bullous pemphigoid

Bullous Pemphigoid is the most common autoimmune blistering skin disease; it is a chronic disorder characterized by the formation of large, tense blisters on the skin surface. It is caused by autoantibodies targeting components of the skin basement membrane [1].

2.4.2 Eosinophilic pustular folliculitis

Eosinophilic pustular folliculitis is a rare skin condition characterized by recurrent episodes of itchy, eosinophil-rich pustules on the skin, particularly on the scalp and face, with eosinophilic infiltration with an increased expression of prostaglandin D synthetase [8] around hair follicles. It is often seen in individuals with HIV infection. The formation of pustules in eosinophilic pustular folliculitis is believed to involve an abnormal immune response and eosinophil activation in the hair follicles.

2.5 Nodular lesions

The nodular patter in dermatoses is characterized by the presence of raised, solid, and rounded skin nodules or lumps. The development of nodular lesions in dermatoses can be attributed to various underlying mechanisms, including inflammatory responses, lymphoproliferative disorders, and hematologic malignancies.

2.5.1 Prurigo nodularis

Prurigo Nodularis is a chronic skin condition characterized by the development of firm, raised, and intensely itchy nodules or papules on the skin surface. The lesions are often symmetrically distributed and may vary in size, ranging from a few millimeters to centimeters in diameter. Itching in prurigo nodularis is thought to be mediated by various pruritogenic factors, including interleukin-31 (IL-31) and oncostatin M, which contribute to the sensation of itchiness and the chronicity of the condition [9].

2.5.2 Cutaneous T-cell lymphoma

Cutaneous T-cell lymphoma encompasses a spectrum of non-Hodgkin lymphomas that primarily affects the skin, including mycosis fungoides and Sézary syndrome, which are the most common subtypes. It may present with nodular lesions, plaques, or erythroderma (widespread redness of the skin) on the skin surface, causing itching that can commonly be severe [10].

2.6 Vasculitis

The vasculitis pattern in dermatoses is characterized by inflammation of blood vessels in the skin, leading to a range of skins manifestation, including purpura, nodules, and other vascular lesions. Eosinophils may be involved in the inflammatory infiltrate associated with vasculitis, contributing to tissue damage and vascular pathology.

2.6.1 Eosinophilic granulomatosis with polyangiitis

Formerly known as Churg-Strauss Syndrome, Eosinophilic Granulomatosis with Polyangiitis (EGPA) is a rare systemic vasculitis characterized by asthma, eosinophilia, and vasculitis affecting small to medium-sized blood vessels. It can affect multiple organs, including the skin, lungs, and nerves. In the third phase of EGPA, skin involvement can occur, presenting as purpuric nodules and other cutaneous lesions [11].

2.7 Fibrosis

The fibrosis pattern in dermatoses is characterized by the excessive accumulation of fibrous tissue on the skin, leading to thickening, hardening, and loss of elasticity. Eosinophils have the capacity to induce tissue remodeling and fibrosis in the skin through the release of profibrotic factors and interactions with other cells.

2.7.1 Eosinophilic fasciitis

Eosinophilic fasciitis is a rare condition characterized by inflammation and thickening of the fascia, the connective tissue that surrounds muscles, nerves, and blood vessels, resulting in skin induration and fibrosis. It primarily affects the arms and legs. Eosinophils are often found in increased numbers in the affected tissues and peripheral blood during the early stages, with elevated IL-5 levels [12].

3. Eosinophils on CNS (including eyes)

3.1 Central and peripheral nervous system

Eosinophilic meningoencephalitis/Eosinophilic meningitis has been associated to various parasite infections like Angiostrongylus, Gnathostoma, and Neurocysticercosis, as well as some fungi like *Coccidioides immitis.* Nevertheless, there are some noninfectious causes like lymphomas, medications, and hypereosinophilic syndrome. This entity is demarcated by the quantity of eosinophils in the cerebrospinal fluid with at least 10 or more eosinophils/microL or at least the 10% of the liquid [13].

3.2 Eyes

Allergic conjunctivitis is one of the most common conditions patients refer to the ophthalmologist; the causes may vary including air pollution, pollen, contact, pet hair, atopy, dust, and mold, among others. The histopathology may show similar findings with increased mast and eosinophils [14].

4. Eosinophils on gastrointestinal system

Eosinophils play a crucial role in the gastrointestinal tract, contributing to both immune defense and tissue homeostasis. Eosinophils specialize in defending the gastrointestinal tract against helminth parasites through the deployment of cytotoxic proteins and bioactive molecules, neutralizing and eliminating these intruders, reinforcing the body's immune response in this critical area [15]. Moreover, eosinophils play vital roles in intestinal health by regulating tissue balance and influencing neuro-immune interactions. They maintain gut barrier function, modulate mucosal immunity, and communicate with various cell types through diverse receptors and stored molecules. Emerging evidence suggests their involvement in brain–gut interaction disorders, highlighting their importance in both physiological and pathological processes within the gastrointestinal environment [16].

4.1 Allergic diseases

Patients with allergic diseases may experience gastrointestinal symptoms associated with eosinophilic inflammation. In food allergies, eosinophils migrate into the gastrointestinal mucosa following exposure to food allergens, playing a role in the development of allergic inflammation, resulting in symptoms like abdominal pain, diarrhea, nausea, and vomiting [15]. The prevalence of IgE-mediated food allergy varies between 25% and nearly 70%, with common implicated foods including milk, wheat, soy, egg, nuts, and shellfish [17].

4.2 Primary eosinophilic gastrointestinal diseases

Eosinophils play a key role in the pathogenesis of primary eosinophilic gastrointestinal diseases, such as eosinophilic esophagitis. These conditions are characterized by eosinophilic infiltration in the gastrointestinal tract, leading to tissue damage caused by inflammatory mediators, cytokines, and chemokines [15]. Some differential diagnoses for primary eosinophilic diseases in the gastrointestinal tract include parasitic or bacterial infections, long-standing drug hypersensitivity, inflammatory bowel disease, and hypereosinophilic syndrome.

4.2.1 Eosinophilic esophagitis

Eosinophilic Esophagitis (EE) is a chronic inflammatory disorder characterized by eosinophilic infiltration in the esophagus, leading to symptoms such as dysphagia, food impaction, and reflux-like symptoms [16]. EE impacts people of diverse ages and ethnic backgrounds, with prevalence rates differing worldwide, with annual incidence rates in adults between 2 and 6 per 100,000 individuals [18]. Familial patterns indicate a genetic predisposition toward EE. Diagnosis of EE typically involves a combination of clinical symptoms, endoscopic findings (such as esophageal rings, furrows, and white plaques), and histological evidence of eosinophilic infiltration in the esophageal tissue [17], with at least 15 observed in one high-power field (HPF) of the esophageal epithelium. These eosinophils extend into the lamina propria and submucosa, with the potential presence of cytotoxic proteins.

4.2.2 Eosinophilic gastritis

Eosinophilic Gastritis (EG) typically manifests through symptoms like abdominal pain, nausea, vomiting, early satiety, weight loss, and occasionally gastrointestinal bleeding, often accompanied by indications of food allergies or intolerances. Endoscopic assessment may reveal mucosal features like erythema, nodularity, friability, and occasionally erosions or ulcers [17]. Histological examination of gastric biopsies confirms diagnosis by identifying elevated eosinophil levels in the gastric mucosa, with a diagnostic threshold of $\geq$30 eosinophils per HPF in $\geq$5 HPF [19].

4.2.3 Eosinophilic enteritis

Eosinophilic Enteritis (EEn) may be subdivided into eosinophilic duodenitis, jejunitis, and ileitis. EEn presents with symptoms like abdominal pain, diarrhea, bloating, malabsorption, and weight loss, often accompanied by signs of food allergies or intolerances. Endoscopic assessment may reveal mucosal features such as erythema, edema, and occasional ulcerations. Suggested cutoff numbers for the histological diagnosis of EEn have been established, yet they are not formal diagnostic criteria, with a threshold of ≥52 eosinophils per HPF in the duodenum and ≥ 56 per HPF in ileum [20]. Treatment strategies for EEn parallel those for eosinophilic gastritis, involving dietary adjustments and pharmacological interventions aimed at reducing eosinophilic inflammation and managing symptoms [17].

4.2.4 Eosinophilic colitis

Eosinophilic Colitis (EC) is a rare gastrointestinal disorder that typically presents with symptoms including abdominal pain, diarrhea, rectal bleeding, weight loss, and occasionally features of bowel obstruction, alongside nonspecific gastrointestinal symptoms like bloating and changes in bowel habits. It often occurs in young patients, particularly in infancy, and during adolescence and early adulthood. Diagnosis involves histological examination of colonic biopsies, revealing an increased eosinophil count in the colonic mucosa, and although precise diagnostic criteria are not formally established, suggested cutoff numbers include ≥100 eosinophils per HPF in right colon, ≥84 per HPF in transverse and descending colon, and ≥ 64 per HPF in rectosigmoid colon [20]. Treatment approaches include dietary modifications, corticosteroids, and targeted biologic therapies [17].

4.3 Functional gastrointestinal disorders

Function gastrointestinal disorders (FGIDs) are characterized by chronic or recurrent gastrointestinal symptoms without an identifiable structural or biochemical cause. Eosinophils are implicated in common FGIDs, such as irritable bowel syndrome (IBS), functional dyspepsia, abdominal pain syndrome, and bloating, significantly impacting patients' quality of life by presenting symptoms like abdominal discomfort, altered bowel habits, and bloating. The eosinophil-mast cell axis may play a significant role in FGIDs, affecting enteric nerve function and gastrointestinal physiology. Treatment strategies for FGIDs often integrate dietary adjustments, stress management, behavioral therapies, and medications [15].

5. Eosinophils on genitourinary system

The specific physiological role of eosinophils in the genitourinary system is yet not fully understood, being often an incidental finding on biopsies.

5.1 End-stage kidney disease (ESKD)

Eosinophils play a puzzling role in kidney disease, often appearing incidentally on kidney biopsies. Both blood and renal biopsy tissue eosinophilia are linked to various immune and nonimmune kidney conditions, yet their significance remains unclear. In the context of End-Stage Kidney Disease (ESKD), peripheral eosinophilia has been established as an independent predictor of renal tissue eosinophilia, with subsequent progression to ESKD [21].

5.2 Eosinophilic cystitis

Eosinophilic cystitis is a rare form of interstitial cystitis; it presents with recurrent episodes of urinary frequency, dysuria, gross hematuria, and suprapubic pain during micturition. Its origin is presumed to be immunological, with several predisposing factors including allergies, trauma, parasitic infections, and drugs, though its exact cause remains unknown. It affects individuals of all ages, with a notable predominance in females. Histologically, it is characterized by eosinophilic infiltration of the bladder wall in the acute phase, with infiltration of mast cells, plasma cells, and fibrosis of the mucosa in the chronic phase, creating a pseudotumoral mass that can be mistaken for malignancy on ultrasonography or computed tomography scan [22, 23].

6. Eosinophils on cardiovascular system

Eosinophils are essential for maintaining cardiac homeostasis, contributing to various protective mechanisms. They exhibit cardioprotective effects post-myocardial infarction, shielding against cardiac dysfunction and fibrosis. Moreover, eosinophils modulate inflammatory responses by producing eosinophil-derived factors like IL4 and mEar1, which are crucial mediators of cardioprotection, inhibiting cell death, fibroblast activation, and neutrophil adhesion in the heart [24]. Various pathologic entities, however, including hypersensitivity reactions, rheumatological diseases, and hypereosinophilic syndrome, can contribute to severe eosinophilia, tissue damage, and subsequent cardiac complications [25].

6.1 Eosinophilic myocarditis

Eosinophilic Myocarditis (EM) is characterized by inflammation of the heart muscle due to eosinophil infiltration. EM usually presents with an associated systemic disorder, such as hypersensitivity reactions, immune-mediated disorders, infections, and cancer; in around a quarter of patients, however, peripheral eosinophilia may be absent [26]. In the acute phase, eosinophils infiltrate the cardiac tissue, degranulate, and release cationic proteins, leading to necrosis of the myocardial cells. Chronic eosinophilic infiltration, and subsequent repair of this damage, results in fibrosis of the myocardial tissue. This can mimic acute coronary syndrome and lead to symptoms such as chest pain, shortness of breath, electrocardiogram abnormalities, and heart failure. Diagnosis often involves cardiac imaging techniques like cardiac magnetic resonance imaging (MRI) and endomyocardial biopsy to reveal the infiltrative nature of eosinophils in the myocardium [25, 27].

6.2 Eosinophilic coronary periarteritis

Eosinophilic Coronary Periarteritis is a rare inflammatory condition characterized by isolated eosinophilic injury to the epicardial coronary arteries. Histologically, it shows significant eosinophilic infiltration in the adventitial layer; severe cases show fibrin thrombi and endothelial denudation. Patients may present with chest pain, shortness of breath, vasospastic angina, and, in severe cases, cardiac arrest, even without traditional risk factors. The prognosis is related to the severity of cardiac injuries and the underlying cause of eosinophilia. Treatment may involve anti-inflammatory therapies and, in severe cases, surgical intervention or heart transplantation [28].

6.3 Hypereosinophilic syndrome

Hypereosinophilic Syndrome (HES) is a heterogeneous group of rare disorders characterized by persistently elevated eosinophil levels in the blood (>1500/mm^3) for over 6 months, causing tissue damage and organ dysfunction. Clinical manifestations may range from fatigue to life-threatening endomyocardial fibrosis and thromboembolic events. Classified into variants like lymphocytic and myeloproliferative, HES presents with diverse symptoms including fatigue, fever, chest pain, and dyspnea. Eosinophilic myocarditis can be a manifestation of HES, causing complications such as heart failure and thromboembolic events. Diagnosis involves clinical evaluation, blood tests, imaging, and possibly endomyocardial biopsy. Treatment focuses on reducing eosinophil levels and symptom control through corticosteroids, immunosuppressants, and targeted therapies [25, 29].

6.4 Löffler's endocarditis

Also known as eosinophilic endomyocardial fibrosis, Löffler's Endocarditis is a rare form of restrictive cardiomyopathy characterized by eosinophilic infiltration of the endocardium and myocardium, leading to fibrosis and thickening of the heart valves and chambers. It is considered a frequent complication of hypereosinophilic syndrome, causing tissue damage, fibrosis, and thrombus formation within the heart. This condition can lead to heart failure and other cardiac complications. Diagnosis often involves endomyocardial biopsy to confirm the presence of eosinophilic infiltrates [25, 30].

7. Eosinophils on endocrine system

In the context of the endocrine system, the exact role of eosinophils is not well described. In endocrine organs, eosinophils and their mediators play a role in various reactive states such as infections and chronic inflammatory disorders. Moreover, eosinophils can be influenced by the production of corticosteroids; a decrease in corticosteroids levels, which occur in conditions such as Addison's disease or adrenal hemorrhage, may lead to an increase of eosinophils in the bloodstream [31].

8. Eosinophils on respiratory system

Eosinophils play a central role in inflammation and allergic processes, particularly in the respiratory system, being often involved in more commonly encountered diseases, such as asthma and allergic responses in the upper respiratory tract. Moreover, eosinophils are implicated in the pathophysiology of respiratory virus infections and hypersensitivity responses to viral vaccines, promoting bronchoconstriction and wheezing. Particularly involved in the immune response to allergens, eosinophils are recruited to the airways in response to allergen exposure, further exacerbating allergic inflammation and asthma symptoms [32, 33].

8.1 Asthma

Asthma is a chronic respiratory condition, characterized by inflammation and constriction of the airways, leading to symptoms such as wheezing, shortness of breath, chest tightness, and coughing. It is caused by inflammation driven by various immune cells in response to various triggers (allergens, irritants, infections, and exercise), resulting in airway hyperresponsiveness and remodeling. Eosinophilic Asthma is a type of asthma that is characterized by high levels of eosinophils in the blood, lung tissues, and mucus; other types include non-eosinophilic asthma and exercise-induced bronchoconstriction [32, 34].

8.2 Eosinophilic pneumonia

Eosinophilic pneumonia is characterized by eosinophil interstitial and alveolar infiltration in the lungs and can be divided in two main types: Acute Eosinophilic Pneumonia (AEP) and Chronic Eosinophilic Pneumonia (CEP). AEP progresses rapidly with respiratory failure and diffuse infiltrates, while CEP presents with subacute or chronic symptoms with peripheral infiltrates, both often associated with hypersensitivity reactions, asthma, or atopy. Other triggers include recent smoking cessation, viral infections, environmental exposures, and certain medications. Common symptoms include cough, shortness of breath, fever, weight loss, and night sweats. Diagnosis involves imaging, blood tests for eosinophilia, and bronchoscopy for confirmation. Treatment primarily relies on corticosteroids and may involve immunosuppressants for refractory cases. Managing underlying conditions like asthma is vital for long-term care [32, 35].

8.3 Allergic bronchopulmonary Aspergillosis

Allergic Bronchopulmonary Aspergillosis (ABPA) is a complex allergic lung disease triggered by hypersensitivity to *Aspergillus species* fungus, entailing an exaggerated immune reaction involving T cells, cytokines (IL-4, IL-5, IL-13), and recruitment of eosinophils, leading to airway inflammation and bronchial damage. Clinical presentation often mirrors asthma symptoms with coughing, wheezing, dyspnea, fever, and weight loss. Diagnosis relies on clinical, radiological, and laboratory criteria, including elevated IgE levels, pulmonary opacities, and central bronchiectasis. Treatment includes systemic corticosteroids, antifungals, and bronchodilators. Prognosis is generally favorable, though complications like bronchiectasis and respiratory failure may arise if untreated [32, 36].

8.4 Eosinophilic granulomatosis with polyangiitis

Formerly known as Churg-Strauss Syndrome, Eosinophilic Granulomatosis with Polyangiitis (EGPA) is a rare multi-systemic autoimmune vasculitis involving small to medium-sized blood vessels, typically associated with anti-neutrophil cytoplasmic antibodies. It progresses through stages, beginning with asthma and allergic rhinitis, followed by eosinophilia and tissue infiltration, and finally systemic vasculitis affecting multiple organs. EGPA often involves the lungs, presenting with asthma, often severe, as well as infiltrates visible on imaging, potentially leading to consolidation, bronchiectasis, and eosinophilic pneumonia contributing to lung inflammation. Systemic vasculitis affects lung blood vessels, possibly leading to inflammation and hemorrhage. Pulmonary nodules may indicate granulomatous inflammation, while interstitial lung disease can lead to fibrosis and impaired function, showing restrictive patterns with reduced gas exchange [37].

9. Eosinophils on muscular system

Eosinophilic myositis has been described on three different patterns according to the extent of the affection as focal eosinophilic myositis, eosinophilic polymyositis/ diffuse eosinophilic myositis, and eosinophilic perimyositis. The pathogenesis of eosinophilic myositis remains unclear, although some triggering events, such as trauma or ethanol ingestion, have been proposed.

9.1 Focal eosinophilic myositis

Focal eosinophilic myositis is the most benign form of this condition, considered benign without any systemic manifestations. The definition includes eosinophilic infiltration within one muscle; the inflammation is identified in the perimysium and endomysium, mostly in the lower extremities, with localized pain and swelling [38].

9.2 Eosinophilic polymyositis/diffuse eosinophilic myositis

Eosinophilic polymyositis/diffuse eosinophilic myositis is characterized by generalized myalgia due to eosinophilic infiltration into the muscles and supporting connective tissue structures, being a cause of atraumatic compartment syndrome in severe cases [38, 39].

9.3 Eosinophilic perimyositis

Eosinophilic perimyositis, as the name suggests, only affects the perimysium, not extending into the fascia or the endomysium. The clinical manifestation consists of myalgia predominantly in the lower limbs, similar to other entities, and eosinophils may also be elevated in peripheral blood levels [39].

9.4 Eosinophilic fasciitis

Also known as Shulman syndrome, Eosinophilic Fasciitis is a rare autoimmune disease with an unclear etiology. The clinical presentation involves progressive thickening of the muscular fascia and subcutaneous soft tissue, accompanied by pain and swelling of the extremities. Biopsy will demonstrate an infiltrate of lymphocytes, plasma cells, histiocytes, and, in early stages, eosinophils [40].

10. Conclusion

In conclusion, the eosinophils play an essential role in many diseases, so it is really important to be aware of their impact and how they may affect each organ and system.

Acknowledgements

The authors acknowledge the use of Grammarly for the language polishing of the manuscript.

Conflict of interest

The authors declare no conflict of interest.

Author details

Rosario Medellin-Vallejo* and Barbara Saenz-Ibarra
Department of Anatomic Pathology and Cytopathology, University Hospital "Jose Eleuterio Gonzalez", Monterrey, Nuevo Leon, Mexico

*Address all correspondence to: rc.medellin@hotmail.com

References

[1] Radonjic-Hoesli S, Brüggen MC, Feldmeyer L, Simon HU, Simon D. Eosinophils in skin diseases [internet]. In: Seminars in Immunopathology. Vol. 43. Springer Science and Business Media LLC; 2021. pp. 393-409. DOI: 10.1007/s00281-021-00868-7

[2] Roduit C, Frei R, Depner M, Karvonen AM, Renz H, Braun-Fahrländer C, et al. Phenotypes of atopic dermatitis depending on the timing of onset and progression in childhood [internet]. In: JAMA Pediatrics. Vol. 171. American Medical Association (AMA); 2017. p. 655. DOI: 10.1001/jamapediatrics.2017.0556

[3] Simon D, Wollenberg A, Renz H, Simon HU. Atopic dermatitis: Collegium Internationale Allergologicum (CIA) update 2019 [internet]. International Archives of Allergy and Immunology. 2019;**178**:207-218. DOI: 10.1159/000497383

[4] Pichler WJ. Delayed drug hypersensitivity reactions [internet]. Annals of Internal Medicine. 2003;**139**:683. DOI: 10.7326/0003-4819-139-8-200310210-00012

[5] Musette P, Janela B. New insights into drug reaction with eosinophilia and systemic symptoms pathophysiology [internet]. Frontiers in Medicine. 2017;**4**:179. DOI: 10.3389/fmed.2017.00179

[6] Cugno M, Marzano AV, Tedeschi A, Fanoni D, Venegoni L, Asero R. Expression of tissue factor by eosinophils in patients with chronic urticaria [internet]. International Archives of Allergy and Immunology. 2008;**148**:170-174. DOI: 10.1159/000155748

[7] Altrichter S, Frischbutter S, Fok JS, Kolkhir P, Jiao Q, Skov PS, et al. The role of eosinophils in chronic spontaneous urticaria [internet]. Journal of Allergy and Clinical Immunology. 2020;**145**:1510-1516. DOI: 10.1016/j.jaci.2020.03.005

[8] Nakahigashi K, Doi H, Otsuka A, Hirabayashi T, Murakami M, Urade Y, et al. PGD2 induces eotaxin-3 via PPARγ from sebocytes: A possible pathogenesis of eosinophilic pustular folliculitis [internet]. Journal of Allergy and Clinical Immunology. 2012;**129**:536-543. DOI: 10.1016/j.jaci.2011.11.034

[9] Rüdrich U, Gehring M, PapakonstantinouE,IllerhausA,EngmannJ, Kapp A, et al. Eosinophils are a major source of interleukin-31 in bullous pemphigoid [internet]. Acta Dermato Venereologica. 2018;**98**:766-771. DOI: 10.2340/00015555-2951

[10] Terhorst-Molawi D, Lohse K, Ginter K, Puhl V, Metz M, Hu M, et al. Mast cells and tryptase are linked to itch and disease severity in mycosis fungoides: Results of a pilot study [internet]. Frontiers in Immunology. 2022;**13**:930979. DOI: 10.3389/fimmu.2022.930979

[11] Manka LA, Guntur VP, Denson JL, Dunn RM, Dollin YT, Strand MJ, et al. Efficacy and safety of reslizumab in the treatment of eosinophilic granulomatosis with polyangiitis [internet]. Annals of Allergy, Asthma & Immunology. 2021;**126**:696-701.e1. DOI: 10.1016/j.anai.2021.01.035

[12] Ihn H. Eosinophilic fasciitis: From pathophysiology to treatment [internet]. Allergology International. 2019;**68**:437-439. DOI: 10.1016/j.alit.2019.03.001

[13] Re VL III, Gluckman SJ. Eosinophilic meningitis. The American Journal of Medicine. 2003;**114**(3):217-223. DOI: 10.1016/s0002-9343(02)01495-x

[14] Baab S, Le PH, Gurnani B, et al. Allergic Conjunctivitis. Treasure Island (FL): StatPearls Publishing; 2024; Available from: https://www.ncbi.nlm.nih.gov/books/NBK448118/

[15] Powell N, Walker MM, Talley NJ. Gastrointestinal eosinophils in health, disease, and functional disorders [internet]. Nature Reviews Gastroenterology & Hepatology. 2010;**7**:146-156. DOI: 10.1038/nrgastro.2010.5

[16] Salvo-Romero E, Rodiño-Janeiro BK, Albert-Bayo M, Lobo B, Santos J, Farré R, et al. Eosinophils in the gastrointestinal tract: Key contributors to neuro-immune crosstalk and potential implications in disorders of brain-gut interaction [internet]. Cells. 2022;**11**:1644. DOI: 10.3390/cells11101644

[17] Rossi CM, Lenti MV, Merli S, Licari A, Votto M, Marseglia GL, et al. Primary eosinophilic gastrointestinal disorders and allergy: Clinical and therapeutic implications [internet]. Clinical and Translational Allergy. 2022;**12**:e12146. DOI: 10.1002/clt2.12146

[18] Yan BM, Shaffer EA. Primary eosinophilic disorders of the gastrointestinal tract [internet]. Gut. 2008;**58**:721-732. DOI: 10.1136/gut.2008.165894

[19] Collins MH, Capocelli K, Yang GY. Eosinophilic gastrointestinal disorders pathology [internet]. Frontiers in Medicine. 2018;**4**:261. DOI: 10.3389/fmed.2017.00261

[20] Collins MH. Histopathologic features of eosinophilic esophagitis and eosinophilic gastrointestinal diseases [internet]. Gastroenterology Clinics of North America. 2014;**43**:257-268. DOI: 10.1016/j.gtc.2014.02.007

[21] Tariq A, Okamato K, Tariq A, Rosenberg AZ, Soliman KM, Ploth DW, et al. Eosinophilia and risk of incident end stage kidney disease [internet]. BMC Nephrology. 2020;**21**:14. DOI: 10.1186/s12882-020-1685-3

[22] Cleva M, Ennio B, Ferdinando B, Massimo V. Eosinophilic cystitis: A case report of a pseudotumoral lesion [internet]. Journal of Ultrasound. 2023;**26**:935-937. DOI: 10.1007/s40477-023-00816-1

[23] Ebel Sepulveda LF, Foneron A, Troncoso L, Cañoles R, Carrasco C, Hornig A, et al. Cistitis eosinofílica: Revisión y reporte de dos casos [Internet]. Actas Urológicas Españolas. 2009;**33**:443-446. DOI: 10.1016/s0210-4806(09)74174-9

[24] Liu J, Yang C, Liu T, Deng Z, Fang W, Zhang X, et al. Eosinophils improve cardiac function after myocardial infarction [internet]. Nature Communications. 2020;**11**:6396. DOI: 10.1038/s41467-020-19297-5

[25] Séguéla PE, Iriart X, Acar P, Montaudon M, Roudaut R, Thambo JB. Eosinophilic cardiac disease: Molecular, clinical and imaging aspects [internet]. Archives of Cardiovascular Diseases. 2015;**108**:258-268. DOI: 10.1016/j.acvd.2015.01.006

[26] Brambatti M, Matassini MV, Adler ED, Klingel K, Camici PG, Ammirati E. Eosinophilic myocarditis [internet]. Journal of the American College of Cardiology. 2017;**70**:2363-2375. DOI: 10.1016/j.jacc.2017.09.023

[27] Zhong Z, Yang Z, Peng Y, Wang L, Yuan X. Diagnosis and treatment of

eosinophilic myocarditis [internet]. Journal of Translational Autoimmunity. 2021;**4**:100118. DOI: 10.1016/j.jtauto.2021.100118

[28] Arai R, Migita S, Koyama Y, Homma T, Saigusa N, Akutsu N, et al. Imaging and pathology of eosinophilic coronary periarteritis [internet]. JACC: Cardiovascular Interventions. 2020;**13**:e151-e154. DOI: 10.1016/j.jcin.2020.05.014

[29] Klion AD. Approach to the patient with suspected hypereosinophilic syndrome [internet]. Hematology. American Society of Hematology. 2022;**2022**:47-54. DOI: 10.1182/hematology.2022000367

[30] Zhang Q, Si D, Zhang Z, Zhang W. Loeffler endocarditis with intracardiac thrombus: Case report and literature review [internet]. BMC Cardiovascular Disorders. 2021;**21**:615. DOI: 10.1186/s12872-021-02443-2

[31] Kovalszki A, Weller PF. Eosinophilia [internet]. In: Primary Care: Clinics in Office Practice. Vol. 43. Elsevier BV; 2016. pp. 607-617. DOI: 10.1016/j.pop.2016.07.010

[32] Eng SS, De Felice ML. The role and immunobiology of eosinophils in the respiratory system: A comprehensive review [internet]. Clinical Reviews in Allergy & Immunology. 2016;**50**:140-158. DOI: 10.1007/s12016-015-8526-3

[33] Schetters STT, Schuijs MJ. Pulmonary eosinophils at the Center of the Allergic Space-Time Continuum [internet]. Frontiers in Immunology. 2021;**12**:772004. DOI: 10.3389/fimmu.2021.772004

[34] Hammad H, Lambrecht BN. The basic immunology of asthma [internet]. Cell. 2021;**184**:1469-1485. DOI: 10.1016/j.cell.2021.02.016

[35] Crowe M, Robinson D, Sagar M, Chen L, Ghamande S. Chronic eosinophilic pneumonia: Clinical perspectives [internet]. Therapeutics and Clinical Risk Management. 2019;**15**:397-403. DOI: 10.2147/TCRM.S157882

[36] Gago S, Denning DW, Bowyer P. Pathophysiological aspects of aspergillus colonization in disease [internet]. Medical Mycology. 2018;**57**:S219-S227. DOI: 10.1093/mmy/myy076

[37] White J, Dubey S. Eosinophilic granulomatosis with polyangiitis: A review [internet]. Autoimmunity Reviews. 2023;**22**:103219. DOI: 10.1016/j.autrev.2022.103219

[38] Fermon C, Authier FJ, Gallay L. Idiopathic eosinophilic myositis: A systematic literature review [internet]. Neuromuscular Disorders. 2022;**32**:116-124. DOI: 10.1016/j.nmd.2021.10.003

[39] Boyajian MK, Roussel LO, Khan G, Stopa E, Bhatt R. Eosinophilic polymyositis: A rare cause of atraumatic compartment syndrome of the forearm [internet]. Journal of Hand and Microsurgery. 2019;**12**:S67-S69. DOI: 10.1055/s-0039-1694288

[40] Lamback EB, Resende FSS, Lenzi TCR. Eosinophilic fasciitis [internet]. Anais Brasileiros de Dermatologia. FapUNIFESP (SciELO). 2016;**91**:57-59. DOI: 10.1590/abd1806-4841.20164683

Chapter 6

Hypereosinophilia in Summary

Asuman Akkaya Fırat

Abstract

Eosinophils are white blood cells. They are found in various cellular arrays. Eosinophils play a role in the fight against many parasitic infections. Eosinophilic asthma, nasal polyps, eosinophilic gastrointestinal disorders, polyangiitis, and eosinophilic granulomatosis are diseases referring hypereosinophilic syndrome. Eosinophil granules participate in tissue healing, damage, repair and restructuring processes thanks to proteins and chemical mediators. Interleukin (IL)-5, IL-4, and IL-13′ play a role in the proliferation, maturation, activation, and recruitment of eosinophils. Eosinophils have receptors for various cytokines, chemokines, and adhesion molecules that allow them to participate in inflammatory activities. In response to stimuli, eosinophils may release a range of granule proteins, including major basic proteins (MBPs) 1–2, eosinophil cationic protein (ECP), eosinophil peroxidase (EPX), eosinophil-derived neurotoxin (EDN), cytokines, and cytosolic Charcot-Leyden crystal protein/ galectin-10 (CLC/Gal-10). Eosinophils participate in a variety of biological processes and contribute to both normal and pathological processes. Improvements can be made in understanding the pathophysiological mechanisms of these diseases. It has led to the development of new therapeutics for eosinophilic inflammatory diseases.

Keywords: eosinophils, hypereosinophilic syndrome, blood cells, chemokines, parasitic infections, allergy

1. Introduction

Eosinophils are cells, often living in tissues, whose function is not fully understood. Eosinophils in peripheral blood or tissues can be increased in a wide sequence in severity from mild to life-threatening, and as a result of various mechanisms. When activated, eosinophils can secrete mediators and substances that can damage tissues and contribute to disease pathology (**Figure 1**).

- Eosinopenia, a decrease in eosinophil blood count

- Eosinophilia, an increase (>500 cells per microliter) in eosinophil blood count. Eosinophils generally constitute less than 7% of circulating leukocytes [1]. A significant increase in the number of non-blood tissue eosinophils in histopathological examination is diagnostic of tissue eosinophilia [2]. Various causes are known; the most common is some type of allergic reaction or parasitic infection. Diagnosis of eosinophilia is made through complete blood count (CBC), but

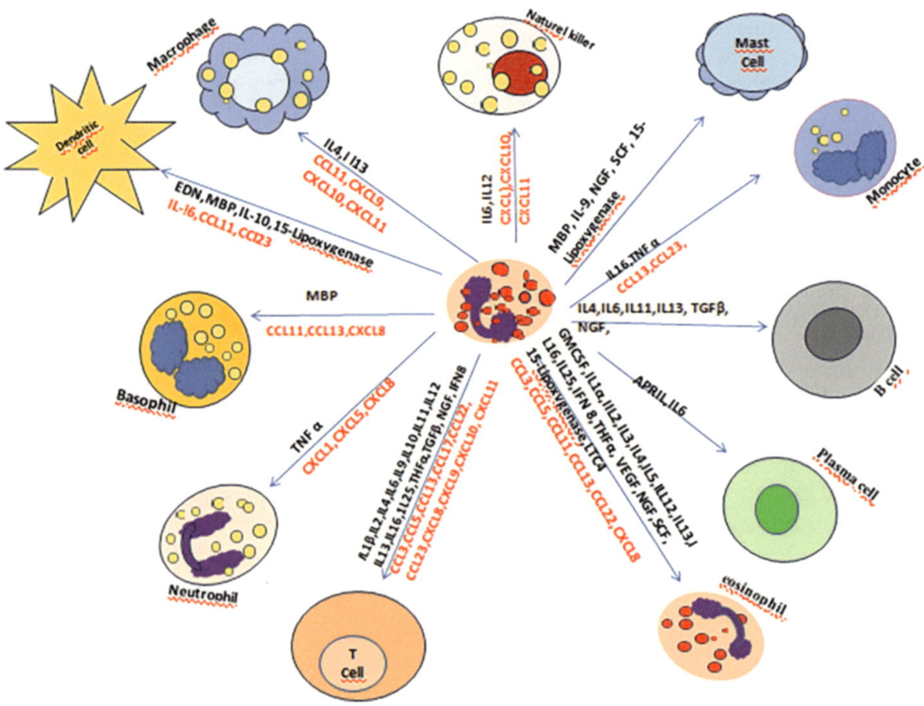

Figure 1.
Functions of eosinophils.

diagnostic procedures for the underlying cause vary depending on the suspected conditions. If the complete blood count shows significant eosinophilia, an absolute eosinophil count is usually not necessary [3]. The location of the causal factor can be used to classify eosinophilia into two general types: *extrinsic*, in which the factor is located outside the eosinophil cell lineage, and *intrinsic* eosinophilia, which indicates etiologies within the eosinophil cell lineage [2]. Specific treatments are determined by the causative condition, but in idiopathic eosinophilia, the disease can be controlled with corticosteroids.

- Hypereosinophilia is characterized by an extreme increase (>1500 cells per microliter) in eosinophil blood count. Hypereosinophilic syndrome (HES) due to overproduction of eosinophils is a disturbance characterized by an increased number of eosinophils in the blood and tissues. Sometimes, eosinophilic infiltration and released mediators may cause damage to end organs. The term HES was coined in 1968 and was introduced by Hardy and Anderson [1–4]. Diagnostic criteria for idiopathic HES were developed by Chusid in 1975. These criteria are as follows:

1. Eosinophilia in peripheral blood is below (>1500/μL) lasting more than a month

2. There is no other cause of eosinophilia

3. End-organ damage or dysfunction

Clonal hypereosinophilia, also called primary hypereosinophilia or clonal eosinophilia, is a group of hematological disorders characterized by the development and growth of a premalignant or malignant population of eosinophils, a type of white blood cell that invades the bone marrow. This population consists of a group of genetically identical eosinophils derived from an eosinophil clone, that is, a sufficiently mutated progenitor cell [1]. The eosinophil clone carries a mutation in any of several genes that encode proteins that regulate cell growth. Mutations cause these proteins to be constantly active, thus stimulating growth in an uncontrolled and continuous manner. The gradually increasing population of eosinophils, which initially forms in the bone marrow, spreads into the blood and can enter various tissues and organs and damage them [1]. Clinically, clonal eosinophilia resembles various types of chronic or acute leukemia, lymphoma, or myeloproliferative hematological malignancy. However, most clonal hypereosinophilias are distinguished from these other hematological malignancies by the genetic mutations underlying their development and, more importantly, by their sensitivity to specific treatment regimens. That is, many types of these disorders are highly sensitive to relatively nontoxic drugs [1, 2].

HES is a heterogeneous hematological disorder. In patient groups with different clinical findings, malignancies belonging to the myeloid or lymphoid series may develop. The development of these disorders suggests that there may be different underlying pathologies. HES can affect both myeloid and lymphoid series. Eosinophils belong to the myeloid series. Clonal eosinophilic differentiation may occur from the myeloid early differentiation stage or from the T-cell series that undergo abnormal differentiation in the T-cell stage. Although demonstrating eosinophil clonality is not easy, it has been revealed recently. An interstitial deletion on chromosome 4q12 leads to the fusion of the FIP1L1 and PDGFRα genes (Fip1-like 1-platelet-derived growth factor receptor alpha). Eosinophil growth factor and apoptosis inhibitor cytokines that cause inflammation are GM-CSF (granulocyte-macrophage colony-stimulating factor), IL-3, and IL-5 [3–5].

Eosinophils are white blood cells (WBCs) of the granulocytic lineage, which also includes neutrophils and basophils. The physiological functions of eosinophils are poorly understood, but they are involved in the host immune response to infection, tissue remodeling, tumor surveillance, and maintenance of other immune cells [1, 2]. Eosinophils develop and differentiate in the bone marrow under the influence of interleukin (IL) 5, IL-3, and GM-CSF. There may be different subsets of eosinophils that play different roles in inflammation and homeostasis [3, 4].

Pulmonary involvement is mainly in the form of chronic dry cough, and infiltration can be seen on chest radiography in <25% of cases. Other target organs where eosinophilic infiltration may be present include the GI tract, liver, spleen, joints, and kidneys. Clinical findings also vary according to involvement. Coagulation system peripheral thromboembolism endovascular damage by eosinophils and peripheral vasculopathy may occur. HES is more common in men than in women (9:1). It is most common between 20 and 50 years of age. Clinical findings vary from patient to patient depending on end-organ involvement. It often has a silent onset, and eosinophilia may be detected incidentally. In some cases, the initial findings may be severe and life-threatening with rapid progression of cardiac and neurologic complications [4–7]. Involvement of the heart, skin, nervous system, lung, and spleen is present in approximately 45–60% of cases. Liver, eye, and GIS involvement is less (20–30%). Directly and independently acts on beige adipocytes via the release of enkephalin peptides. Eosinophils, directly and indirectly, cause blood vessel relaxation in perivascular adipose tissue through adiponectin and catecholamine release, respectively. The catecholamines signal through β3-adrenergic receptors (β3-AR) on adipocytes to cause vessel relaxation *via* nitric oxide (NO) and adiponectin [5–8].

Eosinophilic myocarditis in cardiac involvement is the main cause of mortality and morbidity. Heart damage develops in three stages. The early necrotic stage is rarely symptomatic. This stage is followed by the thrombotic stage with thrombus formation in the damaged endocardium and emboli emanating from it. In the final fibrotic stage, endomyocardial fibrosis and damage to the atrioventricular valves lead to congestive heart failure. Skin manifestations are usually urticaria and angioedema or erythematous, pruritic papules, and nodules. Treatment-resistant mucosal ulcers may also be seen. In neurological complications, the central (encephalopathy) and peripheral nervous system (polyneuropathy) may be affected [6, 8]. The clinical features of different HES subgroups differ. PDGFRα-positive HES occurs almost exclusively in men, often in the heart involvement, and untreated cases have a high mortality rate. In contrast, L-HES does not differ between genders and skin, is prone to soft tissue involvement, and has a rather silent course. Diagnosis in M-HES cases is acute leukemia (eosinophilicor AML), whereas in L-HES cases, there is a risk of developing T-cell lymphoma over a long period [9–11].

2. Diagnosis and laboratory features

Eosinophil count in peripheral blood is >1500/μL. They are usually mature in appearance and rarely can be seen in young cells. White blood cell count >90,000/μL is an indicator of poor prognosis. Anemia may be observed in 50% of cases. Thrombocytosis or thrombocytopenia may be seen. There may be a significant increase in eosinophils and eosinophil precursors in the bone marrow. Chromosome examination is normal in the majority of cases [9–12].

The diagnosis of HES is based on the exclusion of causes of reactive eosinophilia, according to WHO criteria, as reactive causes, infections, hypersensitivity and allergic diseases, immune system disorders, metabolic abnormalities, connective tissue, heart, respiratory system, skin, and GIS diseases. After excluding the causes of eosinophilia, then, at least twice, eosinophil count >1500/μLsymptomatic cases, even in the absence of symptoms should be examined for possible HES. ECG, echocardiography, and respiratory tests should be performed as baseline tests to evaluate end-organ involvement. Chest radiography, and clinical indication, if present, a tissue biopsy should be performed [9–13].

In the third step, the potential downstream of the HES bone groups for the determination of bone cytogenetic examination of marrow, reticulin fibrosis, and special staining for mast cells, lymphadenopathy, and computed tomography of the lung, abdomen, and pelvis should be performed to look for splenomegaly. To these, whether HES is of myeloid or lymphoid origin to establish that it is not. Clinical based on the findings; without cardiac involvement, prominent skin manifestations, high serum IgE levels, or L-HES in patients with hypergammaglobulinemia should be considered [1, 8–12]. Splenomegaly, cardiac involvement, elevated vitamin B12 levels, anemia or thrombocytopenia, and precursor myeloid cells in peripheral blood M-HES should be considered. However, these features are not specific to HES variants, and further testing is needed. This FIP1LI-PDGFRα fusion by FISH or PCR, lymphocyte phenotyping, and T-cell receptor gene reconstitution needs to be demonstrated. Demonstration of T-cell clonal dysfunction for abnormal lymphocyte immunophenotyping, detection of T-cell subsets (CD3- CD4+ and CD3 + CD4- CD8-), or investigation of TCR gene reconstitution by PCR is sufficient. However, in some patients, the etiology is undetectable. This is still a major factor in the pathogenesis of HES [12–14].

Some tests may also help to differentiate between M-HES and L-HES. These include the detection of eosinophilopoietic cytokines (IL-3 and GM-CSF) of the T-cell subset and Th2 (IL-4, IL-5, IL-13) cytokines, and serum tryptase, and measurement of TARC levels is a conventional cytogenetic examination. However, in general, IL-5 levels have no value in classification. High serum tryptase levels or atypical mast cells in bone marrow biopsy cases should be examined for the 816 V ckit mutation for systemic mastocytosis. Conditions that can cause eosinophilia in peripheral blood and tissue may mimic HES. Known etiology eosinophilic diseases (such as helminthic diseases) and those of unknown etiology (Wells syndrome or eosinophilic cellulitis) should be differentiated from HES. One eosinophilic syndrome limited to the organ (eosinophilic pneumonia or eosinophilic gastroenteritis) usually does not show the multiorgan involvement characteristic of HES. Chronic eosinophilic leukemia (CEL), acute eosinophilic leukemia, Churg-Strauss syndrome and systemic mastocytosis with episodic angioedema can be difficult to distinguish from HES [12–15].

Since excessive eosinophil activity can cause end organ damage, the aim of treatment is to reduce eosinophilia. Regardless of the cause and the number of eosinophils (especially in symptomatic patients), the secondary aim is to reduce the damage or the correction. The onset of end-organ involvement is silent and does not always correlate with the degree of eosinophilia. Therefore, monitoring eosinophil count is not sufficient for successful treatment evaluation. Both treatment and follow-up of symptom-free cases, organs, and functions likely to be affected should be monitored. Echocardiography at six-month intervals, pulmonary function tests, and additional tests should be performed. In addition, the underlying disease should be assessed, allowing different treatment approaches to be applied if the disease changes its form [13–16].

Asymptomatic cases with eosinophilia are benign and do not require treatment. In contrast, M-HES, especially in the presence of FIP1L1/PDGFRα mutation, has a highly aggressive course and is fatal without treatment. Therefore, the treatment decision should be based on the patient's clinical and laboratory findings and the results of mutation analysis. For suppression of eosinophilia in FIP1L1/PDGFRa-negative diseases, prednisone (60 mg/day or 1 mg/kg/day) is initially replaced for 1–5 days. This information may be useful if the patient develops rapidly progressive organ involvement requiring treatment. In addition, glucocorticoid response is usually indicative of a good prognosis. Glucocorticoids are the first-line treatment in symptomatic patients or those with end-organ damage. Prednisone 1 mg/kg/day (60 mg/day) may be used in initial treatment. In the majority of cases, it leads to a rapid improvement in eosinophilia and organ infiltration, which leads to the arrest of the inflammatory event and prevents further organ damage. If eosinophilia is suppressed, the dose is slowly reduced and treatment is continued with the lowest dose every other day that controls eosinophilia [14–17].

Hydroxyurea and other chemotherapeutic drugs: hydroxyurea is the drug of choice in steroid-resistant cases, especially in cases of M-HES or CEL. It effectively reduces eosinophil count, improves organ infiltration and hepatosplenomegaly, and delays end-organ damage. An initial dose of 1–2 g is sufficient. The maintenance dose is adjusted according to myelosuppression. Chlorambucil, vincristine, cyclophosphamide, etoposide, 2-chlorodeoxyadenosine, and cytosine arabinoside have also been used in hydroxyurea-resistant, myeloproliferative, and end-organ damage cases. The aim of treatment is the control of organ damage rather than the elimination of eosinophilia.

Cyclosporine A: L-HES is characterized by the proliferation of immunophenotypically abnormal T cells. The release of growth factor by these cells, which stimulates eosinophil-formation, is thought to be responsible for eosinophilia. Some of these cases may respond to T-cell suppressive drugs such as cyclosporin or cladribine. Interferon-alpha: efficacy in some case groups has been reported. It can be used as an initial dose of 1–5 million units/m2/day or 5 days a week. The dose can be adjusted according to patient tolerance. The mechanism of action may be based on suppression of eosinophil differentiation and proliferation. However, in two patients with clonal T cells, IFNa has been shown *in vitro* to inhibit spontaneous apoptosis of clonal Th2 cells [15–18].

Therefore, its use alone in L-HES should be avoided, as it could theoretically lead to the growth of an abnormal clonal community. In addition, in M-HES, imatinib is less toxic than IFNa. A trial of imatinib should be performed before using IFNa. Except for these two patient groups, IFNa is the drug of choice in corticosteroid-refractory patients. Tyrosine kinase inhibitors: the success of the tyrosine kinase inhibitor imatinib in HES led to a search for its target in HES. As a result, the FIP1L1/PDGFRα fusion on chromosome 4 and its product tyrosine kinase were identified. The activity of this mutation can be suppressed with imatinib [16–18].

All HES and CEL patients with FIP1L1/PDGFRA mutations respond to imatinib regardless of disease stage. Clinical, hematologic, and molecular remission is achieved in the majority of patients. Clinical symptoms improve rapidly and eosinophil counts normalize within 1–2 weeks. No improvement is expected in end-organ damage, but it may halt progression. Significant improvement in bone marrow fibrosis is promising. In imatinib treatment, there is a risk of left ventricular dysfunction and cardiogenic shock in patients with cardiac involvement. This has been reported to be reversible with systemic glucocorticoids, intensive support, and discontinuation of imatinib. In patients who are found to have cardiac disease by echocardiography and evaluation of serum troponin levels, it is appropriate to use systemic glucocorticoids (1–2 mg/kg/day) for 1–2 weeks when imatinib is started [15–17]. Some patients without FIP1L1/PDGFRα mutation also responded to imatinib. This suggests that there may be undetected mutations or other targets of imatinib in patients with response. In some patients with no response, the mutation may affect a different PDGFRα fusion partner. As there is currently no test for different mutations, imatinib therapy should also be evaluated in patients with HES with evidence of myeloproliferative disease. Imatinib can also be tried in cases where standard therapy has failed. The appropriate dose and duration of imatinib use have not been established. In patients with FIP1L1/PDGFRα mutation, although it can control clinical symptoms and eosinophilia at a dose as low as 100 mg, it is often higher in patients without mutation. In patients with FIP1L1/PDGFRα mutation, a dose as low as 100 mg can control clinical symptoms and eosinophilia, but higher doses are often required in patients without the mutation. In addition, at low doses, molecular signs of the mutation may persist. According to information from CML, clinical relapse is more frequent if the disease persists molecularly. Therefore, starting treatment at a high dose (400 mg/day) may be a wiser approach [16–20].

In addition, it can be started at 100 mg/day and monitored by fusion gene PCR. If there is no complete response within four weeks, the dose may be increased. In cases where a complete response is achieved but the disease is still present by PCR after 6–12 months, the dose may be increased according to tolerance. Some studies have shown that imatinib is not effective in eliminating early progenitor cells in CML. If this information is adapted to HES, there will be a need for lifelong imatinib use. Serum tryptase level is an indicator of the presence of the FIP1L1/PDGFRα mutation.

It can be useful when genetic testing is not possible. Although primary resistance has not been described to date, there have been a few cases of acquired resistance to imatinib based on a single base change (T6741). Clinical trials are ongoing with some new drugs for the treatment of acquired imatinib resistance. Stem cell transplantation is another treatment modality that can be used in imatinib-resistant cases [18–20].

Anti-IL-5(anti-interleukin-5): anti-IL-5 antibodies (Mepolizumab, SCH55700) have been used in small patient series, and positive results have been reported. No side effects have been reported, and studies with larger patient groups are ongoing. Anti-CD52: eosinophils carry CD52 on their surface. Although response was obtained in treatment-resistant and FIP1L1/PDGFRα-negative cases with alemtuzumab, the disease recurred in some cases following drug discontinuation. Stem cell transplantation: stem cell transplantation, including a reduced regimen, has been used in the treatment of HES in a limited number of cases. It may be useful in treatment-resistant, especially imatinib-resistant cases [18–21]. Findings that may indicate a good prognosis include the following:

- Prolonged eosinopenia on corticosteroid administration
- Elevated serum IgE levels
- Absence of signs of myeloproliferative disease [20–24]

3. Conclusion

Knowledge about the function of eosinophils in health and disease is increasing. Besides their original definition as cytotoxic effector cells, eosinophils are now well-known to be involved in host protection. Eosinophils, immune regulation, priority due to their role in homeostasis and the pathogenesis of allergic diseases may be therapeutic targets. In nonallergic inflammatory diseases, eosinophils represent a breakthrough and are a therapeutic target. Accordingly, eosinophil number and levels are used as biomarkers of many eosinophil-related mediators. Additionally, the prevalence of eosinophils in the tumor microenvironment is associated with outcomes of different types of cancer, and so, promising research continues. Glucocorticoids and monoclonal antibodies targeting therapy mediators associated with eosinophilic inflammation such as IL-4, IL-13, and IL-5 may be a therapeutic target for treatments aimed at reducing eosinophil counts and relieving pain. Emerging evidence suggests that eosinophils have high plasticity potential. Development of new diagnostic and treatment strategies for patients with eosinophilia remains an important requirement.

Abbreviations

Anti-IL-5	anti-IL-5 antibodies mepolizumab, SCH55700
β3-AR	β3-adrenergic receptors
CLC/Gal-10	cytokines, cytosolic Charcot-Leyden crystal protein/ galectin-10
ECP	eosinophil cationic protein
EPX	eosinophil peroxidase
FIP1L1-PDGFRA	Fip1-like 1-platelet-derived growth factor receptor alpha
GM-CSF	granulocyte-macrophage colony-stimulating factor

HES	hypereosinophilic syndrome
IFN	interferon
(MBPs)1-2	major basic proteins
NO	nitric oxide

Author details

Asuman Akkaya Fırat
Sağlık Bilimleri Üniversitesi, İstanbul, Turkey

*Address all correspondence to: asumanfirat44@gmail.com

References

[1] O'Sullivan JA, Bochner BS. Eosinophils and eosinophil-associated diseases: An update. The Journal of Allergy and Clinical Immunology. 2018;**141**(2):505-517. DOI: 10.1016/j.jaci.2017.09.022

[2] Stella S, Massimino M, Manzella L, et al. Molecular pathogenesis and treatment perspectives for hypereosinophilia and hypereosinophilic syndromes. International Journal of Molecular Sciences. 2021;**22**(2):486. Published 2021 Jan 6. DOI: 10.3390/ijms22020486

[3] Groh M, Rohmer J, Etienne N, et al. French guidelines for the etiological workup of eosinophilia and the management of hypereosinophilic syndromes. Orphanet Journal of Rare Diseases. 2023;**18**(1):100. Published 2023 Apr 30. DOI: 10.1186/s13023-023-02696-4

[4] Réau V, Vallée A, Terrier B, et al. Venous thrombosis and predictors of relapse in eosinophil-related diseases. Scientific Reports. 2021;**11**(1):6388. Published 2021 Mar 18. DOI: 10.1038/s41598-021-85852-9

[5] Laurent C, Lefèvre G, Kahn JE, et al. Cutaneous manifestations of lymphoid-variant hypereosinophilic syndrome. The British Journal of Dermatology. 2022;**187**(6):1011-1013. DOI: 10.1111/bjd.21782

[6] Klion AD. Approach to the patient with suspected hypereosinophilic syndrome. Hematology. American Society of Hematology. Education Program. 2022;**2022**(1):47-54. DOI: 10.1182/hematology.2022000367

[7] Diny NL, Baldeviano GC, Talor MV, et al. Eosinophil-derived IL-4 drives the progression of myocarditis to inflammatory dilated cardiomyopathy. The Journal of Experimental Medicine. 2017;**214**(4):943-957. DOI: 10.1084/jem.20161702

[8] Leiva O, Baker O, Jenkins A, et al. Association of thrombosis with hypereosinophilic syndrome in patients with genetic alterations. JAMA Network Open. 2021;**4**(8):e2119812. Published 2021 Aug 2. DOI: 10.1001/jamanetworkopen.2021.19812

[9] Jacobs I, Ceulemans M, Wauters L, et al. Role of eosinophils in intestinal inflammation and fibrosis in inflammatory bowel disease: An overlooked villain? Frontiers in Immunology. 2021;**12**:754413. Published 2021 Oct 19. DOI: 10.3389/fimmu.2021.754413

[10] Tazawa R, Trapnell BC, Inoue Y, et al. Inhaled granulocyte/macrophage-colony stimulating factor as therapy for pulmonary alveolar proteinosis. American Journal of Respiratory and Critical Care Medicine. 2010;**181**(12):1345-1354. DOI: 10.1164/rccm.200906-0978OC

[11] Kuang FL, Fay MP, Ware J, et al. Long-term clinical outcomes of high-dose mepolizumab treatment for hypereosinophilic syndrome. The Journal of Allergy and Clinical Immunology. In Practice. 2018;**6**(5):1518-1527.e5. DOI: 10.1016/j.jaip.2018.04.033

[12] Klion A. Hypereosinophilic syndrome: An approach to treatment in the era of precision medicine. Hematology. American Society of Hematology. Education Program. 2018;**2018**(1):326-331. DOI: 10.1182/asheducation-2018.1.326

[13] Amorim NRT, Luna-Gomes T, Gama-Almeida M, et al. Leptin elicits LTC_4 synthesis by eosinophils mediated by sequential two-step autocrine activation of CCR3 and PGD_2 receptors. Frontiers in Immunology. 2018;**9**:2139. Published 2018 Sep 20. DOI: 10.3389/fimmu.2018.0213

[14] Belfeki N, Ghriss N, Zayet S, El Hedhili F, Moini C, Lefevre G. Successful introduction of benralizumab for eosinophilic ascites. Biomedicine. 2024;**12**(1):117. Published 2024 Jan 6. DOI: 10.3390/biomedicines12010117

[15] Ramirez GA, Yacoub MR, Ripa M, et al. Eosinophils from physiology to disease: A comprehensive review. BioMed Research International. 2018;**2018**:9095275. Published 2018 Jan 28. DOI: 10.1155/2018/909527

[16] Choi JY, Lim JU, Jeong HJ, Lee JE, Rhee CK. Association between peripheral blood/bronchoalveolar lavage eosinophilia and significant oxygen requirements in patients with acute eosinophilic pneumonia. BMC Pulmonary Medicine. 2020;**20**(1):22. Published 2020 Jan 28. DOI: 10.1186/s12890-020-1056-7

[17] Wei X, Li X, Wei Z, et al. Clinical analysis of hypereosinophilic syndrome first presenting with asthma-like symptoms. Annals of Medicine. 2022;**54**(1):11-21. DOI: 10.1080/07853890.2021.2014555

[18] Valent P, Sperr WR, Sotlar K, et al. The serum tryptase test: An emerging robust biomarker in clinical hematology. Expert Review of Hematology. 2014;**7**(5):683-690. DOI: 10.1586/17474086.2014.955008

[19] Sheikh J, Weller PF. Advances in diagnosis and treatment of eosinophilia. Current Opinion in Hematology. 2009;**16**(1):3-8. DOI: 10.1097/MOH.0b013e32831c841f

[20] Roufosse FE, Goldman M, Cogan E. Hypereosinophilic syndromes. Orphanet Journal of Rare Diseases. 2007;**2**:37. Published 2007 Sep 11. DOI: 10.1186/1750-1172-2-37

[21] Diny NL, Schonfeldova B, Shapiro M, Winder ML, Varsani-Brown S, Stockinger B. The aryl hydrocarbon receptor contributes to tissue adaptation of intestinal eosinophils in mice. The Journal of Experimental Medicine. 2022;**219**(4):e20210970. DOI: 10.1084/jem.20210970

[22] Frascoli M, Jeanty C, Fleck S, et al. Heightened immune activation in fetuses with gastroschisis may Be blocked by targeting IL-5. Journal of Immunology. 2016;**196**(12):4957-4966. DOI: 10.4049/jimmunol.1502587

[23] Lombardi C, Berti A, Cottini M. The emerging roles of eosinophils: Implications for the targeted treatment of eosinophilic-associated inflammatory conditions. Current Research in Immunology. 2022;**3**:42-53. Published 2022 Mar 21. DOI: 10.1016/j.crimmu.2022.03.002

[24] Gigon L, Fettrelet T, Yousefi S, Simon D, Simon HU. Eosinophils from A to Z. Allergy. 2023;**78**(7):1810-1846. DOI: 10.1111/all.15751

Chapter 7

The Role of Eosinophilic Inflammation in Inflammatory Bowel Diseases: Conductor or "First" Violin?

Gulustan H. Babayeva, Hikmet I. Ibrahimli, Ferid V. Guliyev, Gunay V. Asadova, Umud R. Mahmudov, Rafail H. Hasanov, Emin Kh. Verdiyev, Jamal S. Musayev, Aychin I. Hasanova, Rashad A. Hasanov, Nargiz E. Afandiyeva, Namig O. Isgandarov and Tunzala A. Maharramova

Abstract

Eosinophils, one of the subgroups of leukocytes, are present in the gastrointestinal tract, with the exception of the esophagus (their presence in quantities of 15 or more is considered eosinophilic esophagitis). Much of the research on eosinophils has focused on their responses against helminths and type II immune system disorders. However, information on the role of eosinophils in the development and maintenance of inflammatory processes, as well as in the formation and progression of fibrotic changes in patients with inflammatory bowel diseases is limited. With increasing interest in innate immunity and the fact that eosinophil granules contain certain inflammatory mediators, eosinophils are becoming one of the current objects of study in inflammatory bowel diseases. In this paper, the authors presented already known data on the functions of eosinophils in inflammatory bowel diseases and some other chronic inflammatory conditions, and also presented the results of their own research on the role and influence of eosinophils on the course of inflammatory bowel diseases.

Keywords: eosinophils, inflammatory bowel disease, fibrosis, gastrointestinal disorders, eosinophil cationic protein

1. Introduction

Crohn's disease (CD) and ulcerative colitis (UC) belong to inflammatory bowel diseases (IBD), are idiopathic heterogeneous diseases, characterized by a relapsing and continuous course [1]. These pathologies occur in genetically predisposed patients as a result of the formation of an inadequate immune response to the intestinal microbiota of the "host" [1]. To date, there is some knowledge about some genetic risk factors, for example, polymorphisms in nucleotide-binding oligomerization domain-2 (NOD-2), the exact pathogenesis unfortunately still remains unclear [1, 2].

In response to the loss of the integrity of the epithelial cover, an excessive immune reaction occurs, which, along with the formation of an inflammatory process, leads to tissue damage [3, 4]. As a result of stable relapse and continuous progression, a similar inflammatory "storm" in inflammatory bowel disease creates the conditions for excessive deposition of extracellular matrix (ECM), leading to intestinal fibrosis (CD is a clear example of this condition). The outcome of fibrosis is the formation of strictures, often leading to intestinal obstruction, one of the most common indications for urgent surgical intervention in patients with CD [4].

According to available literature data, intestinal fibrosis manifests itself only in areas characterized by high activity of the inflammatory process, which once again confirms that an important condition for the development of fibrosis is the presence of inflammation [5–7]. Due to the above, for many years research has focused not on the resulting fibrosis, but on the inflammatory process leading to fibrosis. The characteristics of the main immune components and mediators involved in intestinal fibrogenesis are not fully understood.

Although in recent years the emphasis in the pathogenesis of Crohn's disease and ulcerative colitis has been based more on changes in innate immunity, the main basic research on the pathogenesis of inflammatory bowel diseases has focused on excessive adaptive immune responses [8]. In this aspect, the search for a potential role and "niche" for eosinophils in inflammation and fibrosis has again become relevant [9, 10].

Eosinophils have been identified as important cells contributing to immune cell infiltration in IBD, such as eosinophilic infiltration in the lamina propria in interpretations of the Geboes histological score for UC [11]. It is known that basal plasmacytosis associated with eosinophilia is considered an early distinctive histological sign of the diagnosis of IBD and also closely correlates with histological verification [12]. One of the predictors of lack of response to therapy in IBD is the presence of eosinophilic infiltration in the lamina propria in biopsies from patients with UC [13]. The abundance of mediators found in eosinophilic granules, which play a role in inflammation and/or fibrosis, makes these cells appealing for addressing fibrostenosis in IBD. Thus, they are significant in the quest for new treatment "targets" [8]. Eosinophilic granulocytes have been suggested to be associated with increasing levels of inflammation and the development of fibrosis, but the causative role or mechanism of this process is still unclear [11].

2. Eosinophils and the gastrointestinal tract

2.1 General characteristics

Eosinophils, belonging to the leukocyte family, are a specific type of white blood cell primarily situated in the lamina propria of the gastrointestinal tract [11]. They function as immune cells residing throughout the gastrointestinal tract, except for the esophagus [14].

In response to IL-3, IL-5, and granulocyte-macrophage colony-stimulating factor (GM-CSF), FOG-1 transcription factor levels decrease, while the expression of GATA-1, ID2, and XBP1 transcription factors increases. This cascade facilitates the transformation of pluripotent hematopoietic stem cells in the bone marrow into mature eosinophils [11, 15]. Once stimulated by IL-5, eosinophils are released into the bloodstream. From there, they can migrate into the gastrointestinal tract by binding to specific chemoattractant molecules like ligand 11CC (CCL11, eotaxin-1), CCL24 (eotaxin-2), CCL26 (eotaxin-3), CCL5 (RANTES), CCL7 (MCP-3), and CCL13 (MCP-4), through their CC chemokine receptors (CCR) such as CCR1, CCR3, and CCR4 [16]. Activation of these receptors prompts both the recruitment and activation of eosinophils, leading to the production of various cytokines (IL-4, IL-5, IL-13, interferon-gamma (IFN-γ), etc.) and chemokines (CCL3, CCL5, CCL11, etc.) [11]. When stimulated by cytokines, in particular IL-4, IL-5 and IL-13, eosinophils undergo activation [17]. Eosinophil activation leads to their degranulation, releasing harmful substances like oxygen radicals, eosinophil cationic protein (ECP), and transforming growth factor β (TGF-β) [10, 18]. This process is pivotal in both starting and prolonging inflammation, often in collaboration with other inflammatory cells. Particularly, Th2 lymphocytes, identified by their expression of the membrane receptor CCR3, play a crucial role, as they associate with eosinophils in clusters during inflammation [11]. Eosinophils were thought to act solely as effector cells of the Th2 immune response, but recently it was discovered that eosinophils have their own functions but are closely related to Th2 lymphocytes [11]. In this scenario, Th2 lymphocytes secrete IL-4, IL-5, IL-13, and eotaxins, facilitating the activation and recruitment of eosinophils [19]. Conversely, eosinophils, by releasing IL-4 and IL-5, prompt the maturation of naive Th0 lymphocytes into Th2 cells, and they also activate pre-existing Th2 lymphocytes [19].

2.2 Chemotaxis of eosinophils

In IBD's active inflammation, eosinophils migrate to the gastrointestinal tract and this migration is driven by chemoattractant molecules binding to receptors on the surface of eosinophils. Chemoattractant molecules not only play a key role in eosinophil recruitment, they also partially serve as eosinophil activators [10]. There are several known pathways for eosinophil chemotaxis.

3. The role of eosinophils in inflammation

3.1 Eosinophil activation

When stimulated, activated eosinophils undergo degranulation and release granular contents into the environment. Several such mechanisms of eosinophil activation are known, for example, tissue damage, bacterial and viral infections, binding of cytokines (IL-4, IL-5, IL-13, IL-33, etc.) and some chemokines (eotaxin, RANTES, etc.) [20–22]. This eosinophilic activation is characterized by increased expression of the surface markers CD44, CD11c, CD11b and CD18. As eosinophil activation is already known to be highly dependent on the cytokine milieu, these markers may help shed light on the incompletely understood role of eosinophils in intestinal inflammation [11, 23]. A graphical description of the eosinophil activation pattern is presented in **Figure 1**.

3.2 IL-4

IL-4, a cytokine, is mainly synthesized by basophils, T lymphocytes, mast cells, type 2 innate lymphoid cells (ILC2), eosinophils, and neutrophils [24]. Its crucial

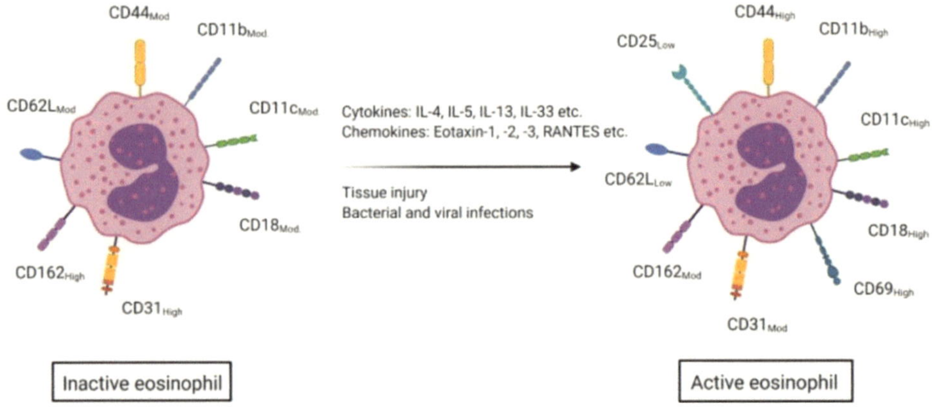

Figure 1.
Eosinophil activation pattern (adapted from Jacobs et al. [11]). Upon contact with certain cytokines (IL-4, IL-5, IL-13, IL-33, etc.), chemokines (eotaxin-1,2 and – 3, RANTES, etc.), as well as tissue damage, bacterial and viral infections, eosinophils are activated. This activation is characterized by increased surface expression of CD18, CD44, CD11b, and CD11c (moderate to high expression). CD25 and CD69 are absent on inactive eosinophils but present on active eosinophils (low and high expression, respectively). On the other hand, CD162 and CD31 are highly expressed on inactive eosinophils but only moderately on active eosinophils, and CD62L is moderately expressed on inactive eosinophils but becomes lowly expressed upon eosinophil activation [11].

function lies in promoting the differentiation of Th0 cells into Th2 cells. As a result, Th2 cells produce IL-4, setting up a "vicious circle" that enhances the differentiation of Th2 lymphocytes [25]. This pro-inflammatory cytokine is known to be a stimulator of eosinophilic transmigration across the endothelium and Th2 lymphocyte differentiation, which also leads to the release of cytokines [11]. By enhancing the expression of eotaxin, IL-4 also promotes the accumulation of eosinophils and their chemotaxis [11]. IL-4 plays a critical role in asthma and allergic inflammation. Its involvement in the pathogenesis of IBD has been extensively studied, where it contributes significantly to inflammation and immune response activation. Increased IL-4 expression has been noted in patients with UC [26]. Research on IL-4 deficiency has demonstrated its ability to prevent colitis development in IL-10 knockout mice, which typically develop colitis spontaneously [11]. Additionally, evidence from models like dextran sodium sulfate (DSS)-induced colitis and the T-cell transfer model suggests that IL-4 may also participate in the development of colitis [27, 28]. A dual IL-4/IL-13 antagonist evaluated in a mouse model of oxazolic colitis was shown to reduce overall disease activity [29].

3.3 IL-5

IL-5 is a chemotactic agent that promotes the differentiation of eosinophils in the bone marrow and may differ in its ability to activate them. During degranulation, eosinophils produce and secrete IL-5, thereby promoting their own differentiation and activation [11]. IL-5 is synthesized in greater quantities by Th2 lymphocytes and ILC2s, and in smaller quantities by NKT cells, mast cells and eosinophils [30]. ILC2 promote eosinophil activation by synthesizing IL-4 and IL-5 (interacts with eotaxins), as well as IL-13 [31, 32]. Specific inhibition of IL-5 attenuates the type 2 immune response and the clinical severity of the disease in patients with eosinophilic asthma, indicating an important role for IL-5 in eosinophil-associated pathologies [33, 34].

3.4 IL-13

The cytokine IL-13 is produced by Th2 lymphocytes, CD4 and NKT cells, basophils, mast cells and eosinophils. Previously, as a mediator of allergic inflammation, it was associated with airway hyperresponsiveness and the development of fibrosis [11]. Due to the common receptor formed by IL-4Rα and IL-13Rα1, IL-13 and IL-4 share certain functional similarities. Activation of this shared receptor initiates STAT6 signaling and supports type 2 immunity. Furthermore, IL-13 can bind to IL-13Rα2, acting as a decoy receptor and thus blocking IL-13 signaling [35].

This cytokine also binds IL-13Rα2 400-fold higher than IL-4Rα/IL-13Rα1, thereby inhibiting STAT6 signaling and attenuating the subsequent type 2 immune response [36]. IL-13Rα2 knockout mice are protected from induction of colitis in a DSS-induced colitis model [36]. However, previous data revealed that IL-13Rα2 knockout mice were not protected from the development of colitis, but recovered rather faster and had faster colonic mucosal repair [35]. Evidence suggests elevated IL13Rα2 mRNA expression levels in mucosal biopsies from IBD patients during active disease, which has been proposed as a biomarker of α-TNF insensitivity [37].

While the exact function of IL-13 in IBD development is not fully understood, there is a possibility that it could be a promising target for IBD therapy [38].

3.5 IL-33

IL-33 is a pro-inflammatory cytokine produced by various intestinal cells, including ILC2, Th2 lymphocytes, and epithelial cells. It interacts with the suppression of tumorigenicity 2 (ST2) receptor present on the eosinophil membrane, thereby activating the ST2/IL-33 signaling pathway [39]. IL-33 is released upon epithelial damage and can independently influence eosinophils, ILC2, and Th2 cells. ILC2 and Th2 cells can enhance the proliferation of eosinophils by producing IL-5 and IL-13, as well as synthesizing IL-4 [40]. Some studies have suggested a potential role for IL-33 in the development of colitis: in UC patients, it was demonstrated that activated eosinophils together with increased IL-33 mRNA expression levels in the colon were correlated with increased eotaxin-1 expression [41]. In both intestinal biopsies from IBD patients and the colons of SAMP/YitFc mice, which develop colitis spontaneously, ST2/IL-33 signaling initiates activation and eosinophilic infiltration. This aligns with a Th2-mediated immune response, facilitating the release of IL-4, IL-5, and IL-13 [42, 43]. Blocking ST2 in these SAMP/YitFc mice reduced Th2 cytokine production and reduced eosinophil recruitment to the ileum [43].

3.6 Eosinophil degranulation

When eosinophils are activated and their subsequent degranulation, various substances can be released into the environment, often characterized by toxicity. According to specific literature, the release of eosinophil-specific proteins such as eosinophil cationic protein (ECP), eosinophil peroxidase (EPO), eosinophil-derived neurotoxin (EDN), and eosinophil major basic protein (MBP) contributes to tissue damage due to their cytotoxic effects. This cytotoxicity results in the destruction of the epithelial layer. According to other data, the TGF-β1 protein released from eosinophil granules also stimulates inflammatory activity and the formation of fibrosis [11].

4. What is the key role of these proteins in the formation of inflammation in the intestines?

4.1 Transforming growth factor β1 (TGF-β1)

TGF-β1 is a cytokine produced by epithelial and immune cells, as well as fibroblasts, and is the most common form in the gastrointestinal tract (compared to TGF-β2 and TGF-β3) [44]. Current literature contains rather contradictory results regarding the role of TGF-β1 in acute intestinal inflammation [45].

4.2 Eosinophil cationic protein (ECP)

Degranulation of eosinophils causes the release of eosinophil-specific ECP, also known as ribonuclease-3, weighing between 18 to 22 kDa. ECP has the ability to harm cell membranes by creating pores in transmembrane channels, facilitating the entry of toxic molecules into the cell. Eosinophils store significant amounts of ECP, which is expelled upon degranulation, eliminating the need for new synthesis during this process [11]. Patients with active IBD had increased serum EPC levels compared with healthy controls or patients with IBD in remission [46]. One study found that an increase in fecal EPC was the same in both CD and UC. However, compared with fecal calprotectin, the diagnostic accuracy was lower in differentiating between active and inactive IBD. However, it was high levels of fecal EPC that correlated with the need for changes in treatment strategy, indicating that this marker can be used as a diagnostic tool to monitor remission in patients with IBD [47]. Moreover, increased deposition of ECP and MBP in the small intestine has been demonstrated in patients with eosinophilic gastroenteritis and correlated with disease severity [11]. Exactly, the evidence suggests a correlation between elevated ECP levels and relapse in inflammatory bowel disease, but further research is needed to determine whether ECP directly contributes to inflammation or if its elevation is merely a consequence of the inflammatory process.

4.3 Eosinophil peroxidase (EPO)

Absolutely, toxic cationic eosinophil peroxidase (EPO) indeed generates hypohalous, bromous, and hypochlorous acids by utilizing hydrogen peroxide, halide ions, and bromide. This process results in the formation of these acids, which have the potential to induce cell damage [48]. Biopsies from the colon mucosa of patients with CD and perfusion fluids from the colon of patients with UC show increased levels of EPO during relapse [49]. EPO causes structural damage by oxidizing nitrates and thus producing toxic reactive oxygen species. These reactive oxygen species have previously been associated with renal inflammation and fibrosis [11].

4.4 Eosinophil-derived neurotoxin (EDN)

Contrary to its name, EDN is not neurotoxic to the human body (neuropathological reactions were detected in a mouse model) [48]. Amcoff K. and his co-authors reported increased levels of EDN protein in the feces of patients with UC not only at the time of relapse, but also 3 months before relapse. Indeed, fecal eosinophil-derived neurotoxin (EDN) has been proposed as a biomarker or predictor of relapse [50]. This prognostic role of EDN in eosinophil-mediated intestinal inflammation has been particularly suggested in pediatric patients [51]. Thus, EDN holds promise as a diagnostic tool or biomarker for gastrointestinal inflammation. However, the question of whether this protein directly contributes to inflammation or fibrosis is still a matter of debate.

4.5 Eosinophil major basic protein (MBP)

Exactly, MBP, also known as proteoglycan 2 (PRG2), is encoded by the PRG2 gene and manifests in two forms: MBP1, which is present in eosinophils, basophils, and mast cells, and MBP2, exclusive to eosinophils [52]. Due to its cationic nature, MBP can disrupt the permeability and function of cell membranes. It is believed that MBP, because of its toxicity, directly increases the permeability of the epithelial layer [52].

Thus (summarized in **Table 1**), eosinophils are involved in the inflammatory process in patients with inflammatory bowel disease [10, 11]. Studies demonstrate an increase in the number of activated eosinophils in both active and inactive UC compared to healthy individuals [18]. Since the presence of activated eosinophils was more pronounced in remission of UC compared to relapse of UC, it is assumed

	Pre-clinical evidence	**Clinical evidence**
IL-4	IL-4 blocking in IL-10 deficient mice: protected from colitis development No IL-4Rα: no disease development	UC patients: ↑ IL-4 expression levels in inflamed mucosa CD patients: ↓ IL-4 levels in intestinal tissue due to lower numbers of IL-4 producing cells in mucosal biopsies
IL-13	IL-4/IL-13 dual antagonist in oxazolone colitis model • Reduced overall disease activity IL-4/IL-13 blocking trough a shared receptor • Reduced overall disease severity {IL-13Rα2 KO model • -IL-13Rα2 antibody mediated depletion DSS model: mice protected from colitis introduction • IL-13Rα2 KO model: not protected from colitis development but recovered faster	CD and UC patients: ↑ IL-13Rα2 in mucosal biopsies Potential biomarker for anti-TNF non-responsiveness Clinical trial with Tralokinumab and Anrukinzumab: no therapeutic effects
IL-5		{Mepolizumab & Reslizumab Benralizumab Attenuates type 2 response + used and shown effective in eosnophl eosinophilic asthma patients UC patients' rectal perfusion fluids: • ↑ IL-5 levels
IL-33	SAMP/YitFc colitis model and antibody mediated ST2 blocking: • ↓ Th2 cytokine production and ↓ eosinophil recruitment into the ileum C57BL/6 ST2 KO mice and ST2 antibody mediated depletion in C57BL/6 mice alleviated disease symptoms	UC patients: ↑ colonic IL-33 mRNA levels and activated eosinophils BD patients' intestinal biopsies: • ST2/IL-33 signaling • Eosinophil infiltration which coincided with Th2 mediated immune response • IL-4, IL-5 and IL-13 release
TGF-β1	TGF- β1 deficient mice: spontaneously develop colitis	Active inflammation in IBD patients: ↑ ↓}TGF – β1 protein levels

	Pre-clinical evidence	Clinical evidence
EDN		UC patients: ↑ f(EDN) protein levels during and 3 months prior to relapse: possible prognostic role Suggested as a prognostic marker in pediatric patients
ECP		Active CD and UC: ↑ serum ECP compared to HC Eosinophil gastroenteritis: ECP and MBP deposition in small bowel
MBP	MBP KO mice: no colitis development upon oxazolone exposure In vitro co-culture of eosinophils and epithelial cells decreased functioning of the epithelial barrier • attributed to MBP	MBP directly increases epithelial layer permeability via its toxicity

Table 1.
The role of eosinophil-activating mediators and compounds from eosinophil-specific granules in intestinal inflammation [11].

that eosinophils are also involved in tissue repair and remodeling mechanisms [18]. Moreover, tissue samples from patients with inflammatory bowel disease showed an increase in the number of degranulated eosinophils and the level of eosinophil granules. Peripheral eosinophilia is associated with worse clinical outcomes and more severe UC [53, 54]. Indeed, it has been demonstrated in vivo that IL-4 production by eosinophils contributes to the development of colitis in both chemically induced dextran sodium sulfate (DSS) and T cell transfer models [55]. Although some similar studies have suggested a role for eosinophils in inflammation, conclusive evidence is lacking.

5. The role of eosinophils in fibrosis

Since eosinophil infiltration has already been identified in other diseases with characteristic fibrosis (endomyocardial fibrosis, idiopathic retroperitoneal fibrosis, pulmonary fibrosis, etc.), therapeutic effects on eosinophils may be quite useful in a number of other fibrotic manifestations [11]. Absolutely, the involvement of eosinophils in the development of intestinal fibrosis in IBD is still not fully understood. Therefore, gaining a precise understanding of the mechanism or function of eosinophils in these fibrotic changes requires further comprehensive investigation. We provide a description of the participation of the previously mentioned eosinophil activators and eosinophil granule proteins in the process of fibrosis.

5.1 IL-4

IL-4, known for its ability to induce TGF-β1, stimulates fibroblast expression and the release of inflammatory cytokines, thus contributing to inflammation. Elevated IL-4 expression is correlated with pulmonary fibrosis. While IL-4 has been implicated in idiopathic pulmonary fibrosis, liver fibrosis, and cardiac fibrosis [11], its involvement in the development of intestinal fibrosis remains inadequately understood.

5.2 IL-5

This cytokine has also been studied in various chronic fibrotic diseases, for example, in liver fibrosis, which is the most relevant today [11]. Using IL-5 knockout C57BL/6 mice, Reiman et al. pointed out a significant reduction in the development of liver fibrosis, determined using pathomorphology, and came to the conclusion that IL-5 is an important factor in this process [11]. According to the authors, IL-5 stimulates the response of Th2 lymphocytes, indirectly increasing the level of IL-13, which is a key mediator in the development of fibrosis. IL-5 exhibits both direct and indirect effects on eosinophil-associated liver fibrosis [11]. The significance of such a Th2 response has been demonstrated in experimental models of pulmonary, renal, and intestinal fibrosis [56, 57]. Anti-IL-5 therapy has been demonstrated to reduce intestinal eosinophils and suppress the development of radiation-induced intestinal fibrosis (RIF) in mice, highlighting the importance of eosinophils and IL-5 in RIF development [58]. However, research on the involvement of IL-5 in the development of intestinal fibrosis remains limited, emphasizing the necessity for further studies.

5.3 IL-13

IL-13 is also involved in the formation of fibrosis (fibrosis of the lungs, kidneys, liver and intestines), and has been identified as a possible inducer of airway remodeling in patients with bronchial asthma [59]. IL-13, together with IL-4, is responsible for eosinophil activation and can activate and proliferate fibroblasts [60]. This cytokine promotes pulmonary fibrosis, and an increase in IL-4 and IL-13 receptors on lung fibroblasts was observed in patients with idiopathic pulmonary fibrosis [60]. IL-13 is also involved in intestinal fibrosis. Fibrosis in mice chronically treated with TNBS appears to be mediated by IL-13 through the production of TGF-β1, and blocking IL-13 results in the prevention of intestinal fibrosis [61, 62]. Increased levels of IL-4Rα, IL-13Rα1 and IL-13Rα2 were found in ileal strictures from patients with CD, indicating the possible involvement of IL-13 in this process [26]. Despite its involvement in wound healing, tissue remodeling, and fibrosis, the precise contribution of IL-13 to the development of strictures in patients with Crohn's disease (CD) is not fully understood [36]. Even if anti-IL13 therapy was not able to suppress inflammation in patients with UC, its effect on inflammation and especially fibrosis in CD has not been studied [26].

5.4 IL-33

Activation of eosinophils by IL-33 and subsequent co-culture with intestinal fibroblasts resulted in increased levels of certain proteins and molecules associated with inflammation and fibrosis. This includes IL-13Rα2, the cytokines TNF-α, IL-1β and IL-6, and the chemokines CCL24 and CCL26. The release of these molecules, especially CCL24 and CCL26, may enhance eosinophil influx. Fibroblasts isolated from this culture were cultured with IL-13 and began to produce fibronectin, collagen 1α2 and periostin, which are characteristic signs of fibrosis. Thus, eosinophils may play a dual role in inflammation and fibrosis. There is also an increase in IL-33 levels in ileal samples from children with Crohn's disease compared to healthy children [63].

5.5 TGF-β

Indeed, TGF-β, recognized as a profibrotic cytokine, is involved in fibrosis in multiple organs [1, 11, 64]. It has an impact on various airway structural cells, including fibroblasts, smooth muscle cells, and epithelial cells, and is associated with fibrotic processes such as airway remodeling observed in individuals with bronchial asthma [59]. TGF-β prompts fibroblasts to transform into myofibroblasts, consequently contributing to the progression of fibrosis [59]. In vitro cultivation of mucosal fibroblasts obtained from patients with UC during relapse revealed increased synthesis of TGF-β1 and TGF-β3, while mucosal fibroblasts obtained from patients with CD during relapse showed increased production of TGF-β1 and decreased TGF-β3 production. Elevated levels of TGF-β1 are similarly observed in mucosal biopsies from patients with CD [11, 64]. Given that TGF-β is produced by epithelial cells, fibroblasts and immune cells, the role of eosinophils in this condition is not specifically known [44].

5.6 Eosinophilic cationic protein

As previously discussed, this protein has recently been proposed as a potential mediator of tissue remodeling in patients with allergic asthma and eosinophilic esophagitis [65]. In the lungs, tissue remodeling involves the release of collagen and proteoglycans from interstitial fibroblasts. Eosinophils, where ECP plays a significant role, contribute to this process by producing and releasing TGF-β [65]. ECP also triggers collagen gel contraction and intracellular proteoglycan accumulation, potentially affecting fibroblast activation indirectly [11, 65]. However, conclusive evidence is still lacking, and further extensive research is necessary. Additionally, the precise role of ECP in the development of intestinal fibrosis has not yet been fully elucidated.

5.7 EPO

Absolutely, the association of these factors with fibroblast activation suggests a potential involvement of EPO in fibrosis development. However, definitive evidence to confirm this hypothesis is still lacking [11].

5.8 What factors can influence eosinophil function?

Exactly, neutrophil extracellular traps (NETs), which are composed of a complex network of extracellular fibers primarily made up of neutrophil DNA, are indeed associated with both inflammatory and fibrotic diseases. Similar to what has been proposed for neutrophils, they have been found to be involved in tissue damage in the airways of asthmatic patients, which is of interest in the context of the development of fibrosis [66]. Some studies have found a relationship between intestinal eosinophils and the microbiome. Indeed, previous findings have shown significantly higher eosinophil counts in germ-free mice compared to pathogen-free mice, suggesting that the microbiome suppresses eosinophil proliferation [67]. Furthermore, when germ-free mice were exposed to a complex microbiome, a significant decrease in eosinophil counts was observed [67]. There is evidence that the high presence of eosinophils resulting from helminth infections can lead to tissue fibrosis [11]. The microbiome clearly has a direct influence on the number and function of eosinophils. Because eosinophils are present in the gastrointestinal tract under normally homeostatic conditions, it is believed that they play a positive role in maintaining tissue homeostasis. This occurs by maintaining plasma B cells that produce IgA, thereby regulating the composition of the intestinal microbiota and promoting the development of Peyer's patches. Eosinophils enhance the secretion of intestinal mucus and thus help maintain the integrity of the epithelial barrier. Eosinophils release the IL-1 receptor antagonist IL-1Rα, which in turn inhibits IL-1β production, resulting in reduced Th17 differentiation. Given that Th17 cells are key producers of the profibrotic cytokine IL-17A, eosinophils may exert antifibrotic activity [68].

6. Eosinophilic inflammation through the eyes of a gastroenterologist, endoscopist and pathologist

One of the most "difficult" moments in the diagnosis of inflammatory bowel diseases is the correct interpretation of the endoscopic and pathomorphological picture and the corresponding activity of the mucosal lesion.

And first of all, this affects the issues of eosinophilic lesions of the mucous membranes of the small and large intestine. The most commonly differentiated pathology is eosinophilic colitis.

But before touching on the topic of eosinophilic colitis, it is necessary to clarify some aspects of primary and secondary eosinophilic lesions of the gastrointestinal tract (**Table 2**).

Eosinophilic colitis is an extremely rare inflammatory disease of the large intestine. The pathology is characterized by peripheral hypereosinophilia and swelling

Primary eosinophilic gastrointestinal disorders	Secondary gastrointestinal eosinophilic disorders
Eosinophilic esophagitis	Gastroesophageal reflux disease
Primary eosinophilic gastroenteritis	Infections and parasitic infestations: protozoal, helminthic, fungal and other pathogens
Primary eosinophilic colitis	Drugs (e.g., naproxen, clozapine, rifampicin, enalapril, carbamazepine, gold drugs, interferons, tacrolimus)
Food allergies: • IgE-mediated • non-IgE-mediated	Systemic and autoimmune diseases: • systemic connective tissue diseases (for example, systemic lupus erythematosus, scleroderma, Wegener's granulomatosis, rheumatoid arthritis, periarteritis nodosa, eosinophilic fasciitis) • vasculitis • Churg-Strauss syndrome • Tolosa-Hunt syndrome • transplant rejection reaction Helicobacter gastritis Celiac disease Inflammatory bowel diseases (ulcerative colitis, Crohn's disease) Malignant neoplasms Iatrogenic pathology (for example, induced by the use of drugs, the use of medical equipment and instruments)
Eosinophilic (allergic, food protein-induced) colitis of early childhood	

Table 2.
Classification of primary and secondary eosinophilic gastrointestinal disorders.

of the mucous membranes of the gastrointestinal tract. Typically, this condition is associated with individual allergic reactions and/or autoimmune diseases.

6.1 Symptoms of eosinophilic colitis

The causes of eosinophilic colitis are not fully known. Chronic eosinophilic colitis is extremely rare. It is believed to occur due to an allergic reaction to dairy products, eggs and soy. It is believed that the nature of the disease lies in the individual reaction to food allergies and other autoimmune diseases (bronchial asthma, eczema), therefore, when making a diagnosis, it is first of all important to exclude: infectious pathogens of gastrointestinal inflammation, the presence of parasites.

Pathology can affect one or more parts of the intestine. Depending on the depth of penetration of leukocytes into the intestinal walls, the following symptoms of eosinophilic colitis occur:

- when eosinophils affect only the outer surface of the mucosa, problems with malabsorption begin (diarrhea, steatorrhea, deficiency of vitamins (primarily fat-soluble), and a significant decrease in body weight). Along with the above symptoms, associated problems may appear: iron deficiency anemia, hypoalbuminemia, mineral deficiency;

- if the lesion reaches the submucosa and muscular lining of the intestine, the problems worsen. Complete or partial intestinal obstruction is possible, which is accompanied by bloating, abdominal pain, nausea and vomiting;

- if eosinophils completely saturate the intestinal lining, then ascites occurs, which is accompanied by severe swelling, abdominal pain, flatulence, nausea and other gastrointestinal problems.

6.2 Diagnosis of eosinophilic colitis

The broad clinical picture and rarity of the disease oblige doctors to collect many tests to make a diagnosis. In addition to general data on blood, feces and urine, it is necessary to conduct a morphological examination of the walls of the rectum. This requires a colonoscopy with biopsies taken.

In some cases, additional examinations are possible (irrigoscopy, radiography, CT, MRI, etc.).

The endoscopic picture can often be normal or have nonspecific signs of chronic inflammation. Mucosal erythema, fragility, erosion or ulceration, mucous "inclusions" and/or whitish spots may be detected.

Essential for diagnosis is a biopsy, which reveals eosinophilic infiltration of the colon mucosa. Given the nonspecific symptoms of abdominal pain, constipation, diarrhea, and rectal bleeding, the absence of distinctive clinical findings, and the relapsing course, the diagnosis of eosinophilic colitis should be substantiated by examining a colon biopsy [69–73]. Examination of a biopsy specimen usually demonstrates layers of eosinophilic infiltration in the lamina propria of the colon mucosa, less often spreading to the submucosal and muscular layers. Other histological findings that can be observed in the colon are eosinophilic microabscesses, eosinophilic cryptitis and intraepithelial eosinophils located predominantly in the superficial layers [70]. Multiple biopsies are necessary because not only is the eosinophilic infiltration unevenly distributed in eosinophilic colitis, but the normal eosinophil count usually has a wide range in different segments of the colon, showing a "proximal-distal distribution" of 35 eosinophils in the cecum, decreasing to 8–10 eosinophils in the rectum (high magnification microscopy field ×200) [74]. In addition to counting total eosinophil density, degranulation is assessed as an indicator of eosinophil activation. Degranulation can be observed in routinely stained media and assessed semiquantitatively, but it is unknown whether biopsy trauma may otherwise provoke degranulation of inactive eosinophils. In principle, the process of eosinophil degranulation could initiate cellular damage through mechanisms involving lysosomal, oxidative, and cytotoxic pathways. This damage, if sustained over time, might contribute to the development of localized fibrosis [70]. However, it's worth noting that such fibrotic changes have not been documented in the gastrointestinal tract.

In most cases, only evaluation of a mucosal biopsy is available to diagnose eosinophilic colitis. However, eosinophilic infiltration in this case is also possible in the deeper layers of the colon wall. Thus, in three cases of pseudo-obstruction of the colon in eosinophilic colitis, eosinophilic ganglionitis was detected in the Meissner plexus [75].

Currently, the diagnosis of eosinophilic colitis remains quite difficult due to the nonspecificity of clinical manifestations and the lack of generally accepted criteria for distinguishing the eosinophilic density of the colon mucosa in the upper normal range from a diagnostically significant pathological increase in the number of eosinophils.

If we proceed from the ECCO recommendations of August 2023 (Definitions of Histological Abnormalities in Inflammatory Bowel Disease: an ECCO Position Paper) [76], then there is some data on pathological assessment associated with eosinophils (**Table 3**).

In this document in position 3.4. "Eosinophils" published guidelines for the assessment of eosinophils in biopsy material in inflammatory bowel diseases.

ECCO Position 4.1. [70]

Eosinophils do not define chronic inflammation or acute inflammation reliably in inflammatory bowel disease.

Agreement: 93%.

Type of abnormality	Example
Unequivocally abnormal feature	Crypt abscess Granuloma
Features whose occurrence in normal mucosa is a subject of controversy	Lamina propria neutrophils Eosinophil cryptitis
Increase in a feature that is usually absent or sparse	Crypt branching
Increase or reduction in a feature that is normally present	Plasma cells in the basal mucosa [increase] Lymphoid aggregates [increase] Epithelial mucin [reduction]
The severity or magnitude of an abnormality	Mild, moderate, or severe increase in eosinophils / neutrophils / plasma cells
Presence of a feature that is normal at one site but would be abnormal at another site	Paneth cells in right colon [normal] Minor crypt distortion in caecum and rectum [normal]

Table 3.
Broad categories of histological abnormality [76].

ECCO Position 4.2. [70]

There is no widely accepted definition of a significant increase in colorectal mucosal eosinophils in inflammatory bowel disease.

Agreement: 93%.

ECCO Position 4.3. [70]

Eosinophilic cryptitis is defined as the presence of at least one eosinophil in the crypt epithelium.

Agreement: 93%.

ECCO Position 4.4. [70]

An eosinophilic crypt abscess is defined as eosinophils in a crypt lumen without the presence of luminal neutrophils.

Agreement: 100%.

There is a scarcity of data regarding the typical count of eosinophils in the intestinal mucosa, the precise definition of an eosinophil crypt abscess, [77, 78] and the criteria for categorizing an increase in intestinal mucosal eosinophils as mild, moderate, or severe (**Figures 2** and **3**). Additionally, the significance of focal eosinophil cryptitis

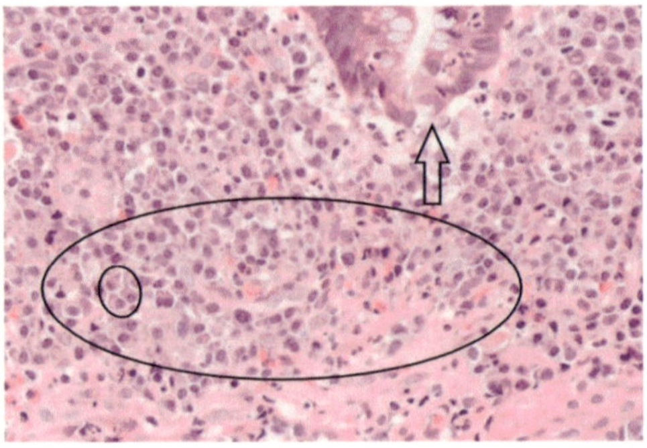

Figure 2.
Basal plasmacytosis, comprising an increase in plasma cell numbers at the mucosa base ['crypts with their feet in pools of plasma cells'] and elsewhere [e.g., within large ellipse; small ellipse surrounds three plasma cells] (adapted Feakins et al. [76]). Other inflammatory cells [e.g., eosinophils] are also apparent. The base of a crypt [arrow] shows cryptitis [i.e., at least one neutrophil in the crypt epithelium] [79].

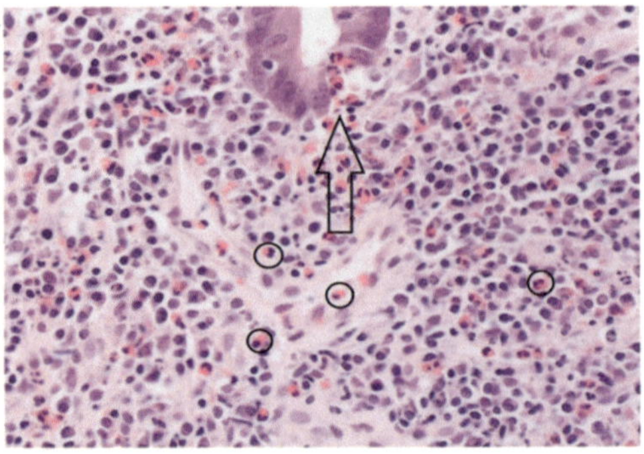

Figure 3.
Eosinophils accompany basal plasma cells in this biopsy [circles identify four eosinophils] (adapted Feakins et al. [76]). A crypt shows eosinophil cryptitis [arrow; ie, at least one eosinophil in the crypt epithelium without accompanying neutrophils]. The maximum number of lamina propria eosinophils and of foci of eosinophilic cryptitis in normal mucosa is uncertain.

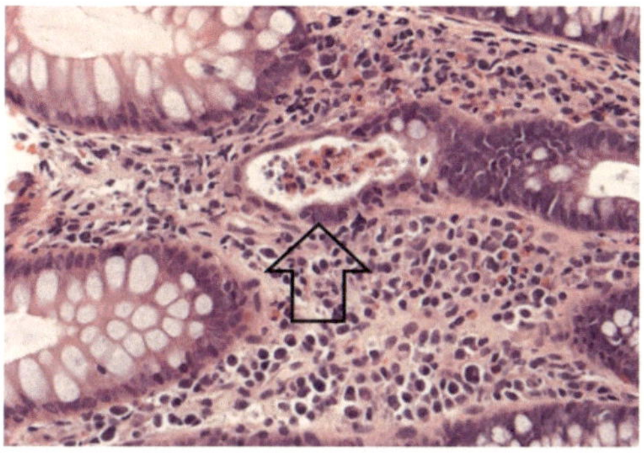

Figure 4.
This crypt abscess [arrow] consists mainly of eosinophils but also includes neutrophils (adapted Feakins et al. [76]). Therefore, it is a crypt abscess rather than an eosinophil crypt abscess.

in the absence of other alterations remains uncertain. The consensus among experts is that an eosinophilic crypt abscess involves the presence of at least two eosinophils. If neutrophils are also present, the lesion is termed a crypt abscess (i.e., neutrophil crypt abscess; **Figure 4**).

To treat eosinophilic colitis and alleviate the patient's condition, different methods are used: the use of medications (glucocorticosteroids, antihistamines, mesalazine, leukotriene inhibitors, azathioprine and biological treatments); a diet excluding allergens is prescribed.

The effectiveness of treatment lies in reducing the density of eosinophilic infiltration, that is, the area of damage to the tissues of the gastrointestinal tract by leukocytes. Therefore, repeated intestinal biopsies are necessary during treatment.

7. The influence of elevation of the level of eosinophilic cationic protein on the course of inflammatory bowel diseases (results of our own research)

We conducted a small study related to the effect of increased eosinophil cationic protein in patients with inflammatory bowel diseases on disease activity.

Study objective: To investigate the impact of elevated levels of eosinophilic cationic protein on the progression of inflammatory bowel diseases.

Materials and methods: The study was conducted between January 2016 and April 2022, involving a cohort of 400 patients diagnosed with inflammatory bowel disease (Crohn's disease (CD): 238 patients, Ulcerative Colitis (UC): 150 patients, Microscopic Colitis (MC): 12 patients). Each participant underwent endoscopic examination with biopsy sampling for histopathological analysis, along with a series of laboratory tests including complete blood count, CRP, homocysteine, vitamin D levels, ANCA markers, α-TNF and IL-1β, IL-2, IL-4, IL-6, IL-8, IL-10, IL-18 levels, total protein, albumin, iron, ferritin, eosinophil cationic protein (ECP), IgE levels, urinalysis with urine albumin, and measurement of fecal calprotectin and lactoferrin levels.

Results: Among the 250 patients (62.5%) exhibiting inadequate response to standard therapy, eosinophilic cationic protein levels were assessed in the blood. Among them, 69 cases (27.6%) tested positive. Notably, 190 patients (76%) demonstrated positive endoscopic findings. Furthermore, 95 patients (38%) showed positive histopathological findings, characterized by the presence of more than 15–20 eosinophils per field of view in the biopsy samples. Additionally, 14 patients (5.6% / 20.2%)

were diagnosed with concurrent allergic diseases. The level of eosinophilic cationic protein in the blood ranged from 29 to 228 ng/ml (N < 24 ng/ml). In the group of patients with elevated levels of eosinophilic cationic protein, the number of patients with Crohn's disease increased (41 patients), including patients with phenotype B2 (24 patients), and patients with phenotype B3 (17). Basic patient data and changes in follow-up are presented in the **Figures 5–7**.

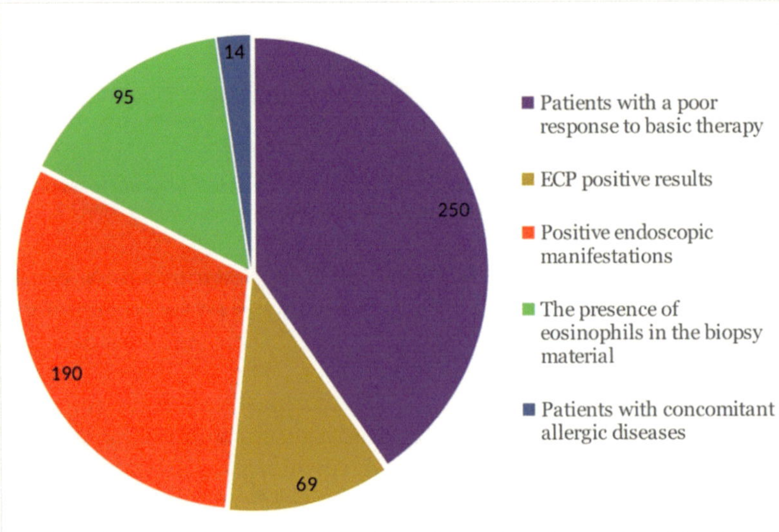

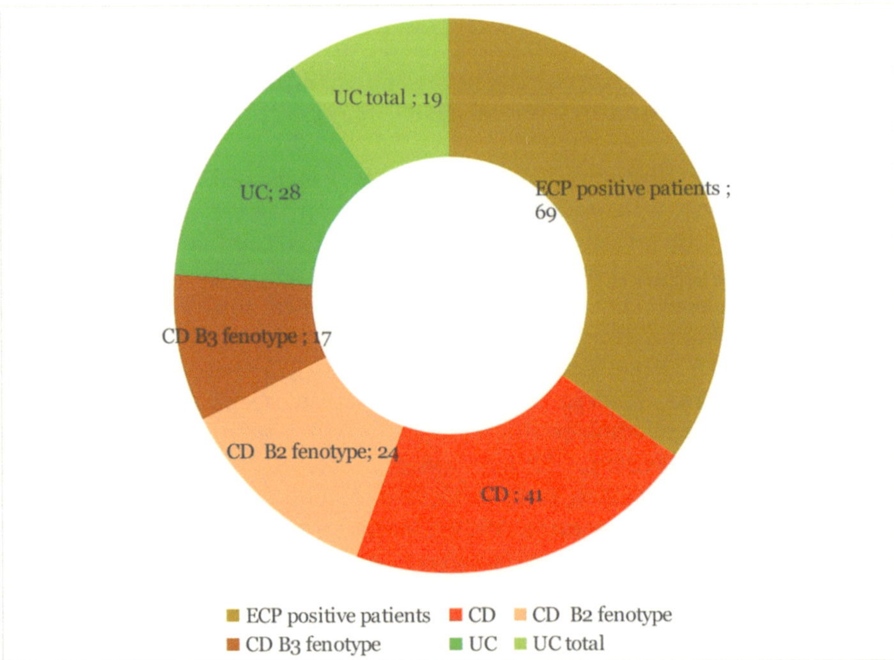

Figure 5.
Distributions of patients. (a) General distribution of patients. (b) Distribution of patients by nosology and phenotypes.

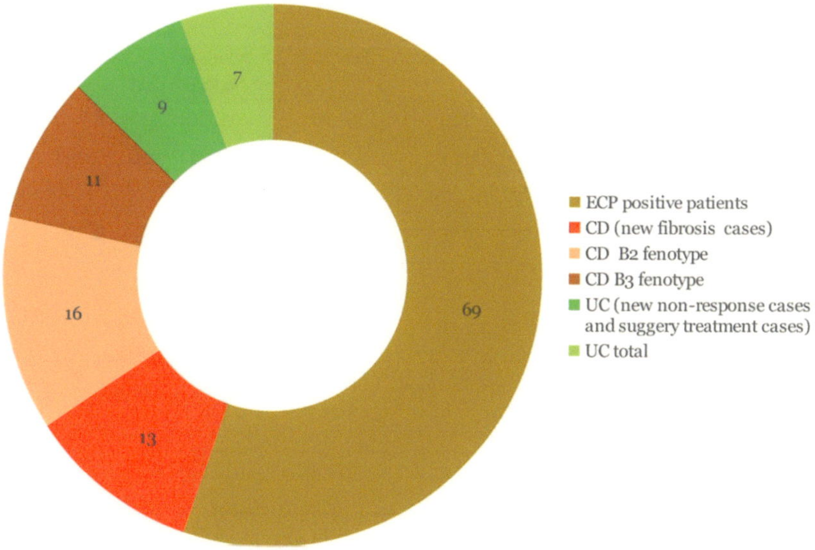

Figure 6.
Distribution of patients after 6-24 months.

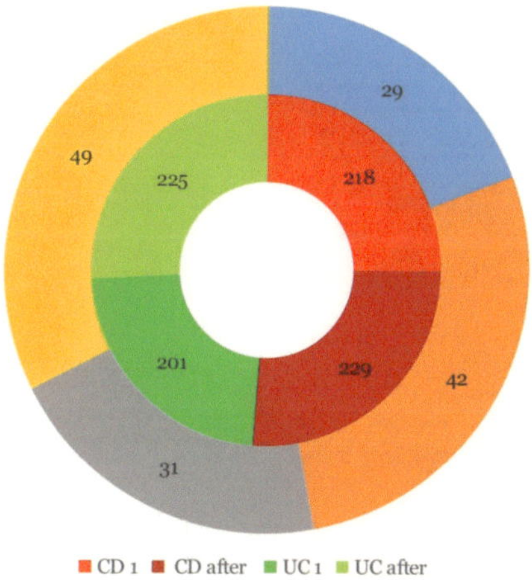

Figure 7.
Distribution by EPC level.

During the dynamic follow-up of patients with elevated eosinophilic cationic protein levels over 6–24 months, several developments were observed. In patients with Crohn's disease, new instances of fibrosis emerged. Similarly, cases of unresponsiveness to standard therapy and subsequent surgical interventions were noted in patients with ulcerative colitis. Importantly, the levels of eosinophilic cationic protein elevation were higher in the group of patients experiencing complications compared to those without complications. The results of some laboratory parameters, indicators of endoscopic and histological activity of the course of inflammatory bowel diseases, depending on changes in the level of eosinophilic cationic protein are presented in **Tables 4** and **5**.

Images from endoscopic examinations (colonoscopy) and pathological examinations of biopsies taken from the mucous membranes of the colon and terminal ileum

Activity indicators	EPC+(N < 24 ng/mL)			EPC-		
	Average value	UC n = 35	CD n = 34	Average value	UC n = 35	CD 11 = 34
h/s CRP (N < 1 mg/L)	16.85	15.1	18.6	6.35	6.9	5.8
Plateles (N 150–400,000/mm^3)	461.65	436.1	487.2	335.75	319.9	351.6
Homocystein (N < 12 μmol/L)	17.05	15.9	18.2	10.25	9.6	10.9
Vitamin D (N 30-100 ng/mL)	4.9	4.0	5.8	20.9	23.1	18.7
Calprotectin (N < 50 μg/g)	1791	2354	1228	1269	1563	975
Albumin (in urina) (N < 2 mg/L)	37.25	32.1	42.4	8.3	10.2	6.4
Laktoferrin (N < 7.5 μg/g)	135.5	144	127	57.5	76	39
α-TNF (N 4.6–12.4 pg./ml)	12.5	12.1	12.9	11.25	10.4	12.1
Il-1β (N < 11 pq/ml)	10.45	10.2	10.7	10.4	10.3	10.5
Il-2 (N < 10 pq/ml)	3.2	2.9	3.5	2.85	2.9	2.8
İl-4(N < 4 pq/ml)	3.85	3.9	3.8	2.25	2.2	2.3
İl-6(N < 10 pq/ml)	8.7	8.5	8.9	8.8	8.7	8.9
İl-8(N < 10 pq/ml)	11.1	10.9	11.3	10.35	10.1	10.6
İl-10(N < 20 pq/ml)	21.5	21.2	21.8	18.75	18.4	19.1
İl-18(N < 261 pq/ml)	265.3	264.5	266.1	252.1	258.4	245.8
Endoscopic activity	++*	+++	++++	++	+++	++
Morphological activity	+++**	++++	+++	++	++	++

**moderate activity.*
***high activity.*

Table 4.
Changes in activity in some laboratory, endoscopic and pathological parameters.

Activity indicators	ECP+ Average value	ECP– Average value
Total protein (N 66–87q/l)	62.1	74.3
Albumen (N 35–52 g/L)	29.3	39.7
Iron (N 27–150 μg/dL)	10.8	46.1
Ferritin (N 10–154 ng/mL)	7.5	62.7
IgE (N < 100 IU/mL)	89.6	67.3

Table 5.
Changes in total protein, albumin, iron, ferritin, IgE.

in patients with elevated blood levels of eosinophil cationic protein are presented in **Figures 8** and **9** (the presentedmaterials are archival data of doctors Gulustan H. Babayeva, Gunay V. Asadova, Jamal S. Musayev).

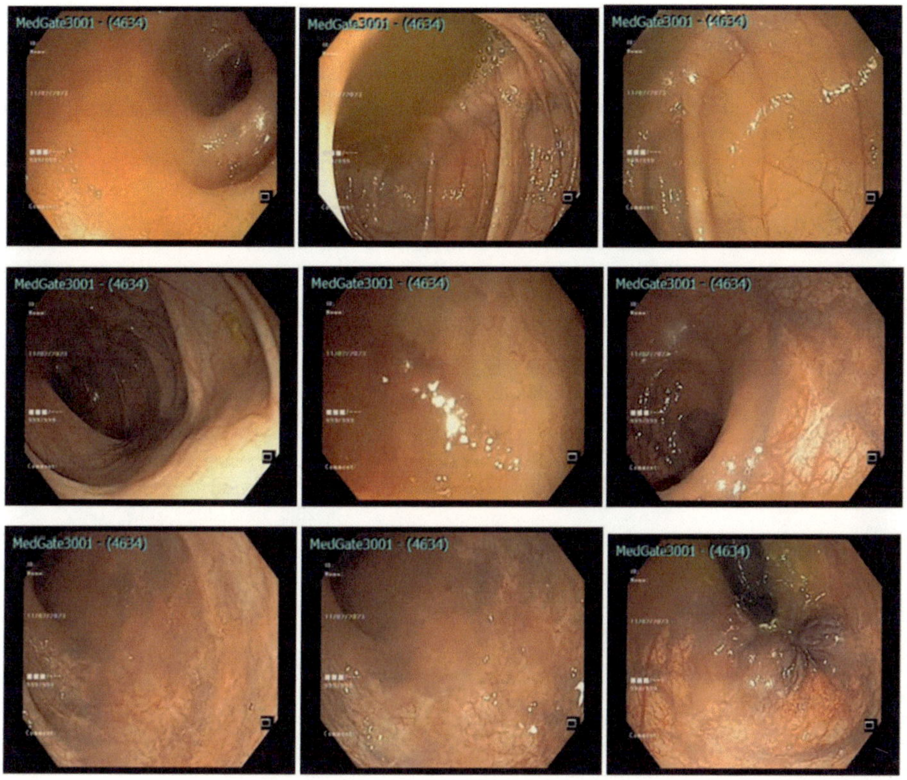

Figure 8.
Patient C.E.N., male, born in 1988. She has been ill since 2018; in 2019, the diagnosis of Crohn's disease (L3, B2, narrowing in the area of the terminal ileum) was verified. (a) Data from endoscopic examination of the colon and terminal ileum. Endoscopic conclusion: Terminal ileitis. Inflammatory bowel disease with ulcerative lesions of the periappendicular and rectosigmoid areas, high endoscopic activity, subcompensated stenosis (Crohn's disease). (b) Data from a pathomorphological study of a biopsy taken from the mucous membrane of the colon. Conclusion of the pathomorphological study: against the background of swelling and ulcerative defect of the colon mucosa, lymphocytes, plasma cells and eosinophilic infiltration were detected in the lamina propria (over 60-65 eosinophils per 1 HPF).

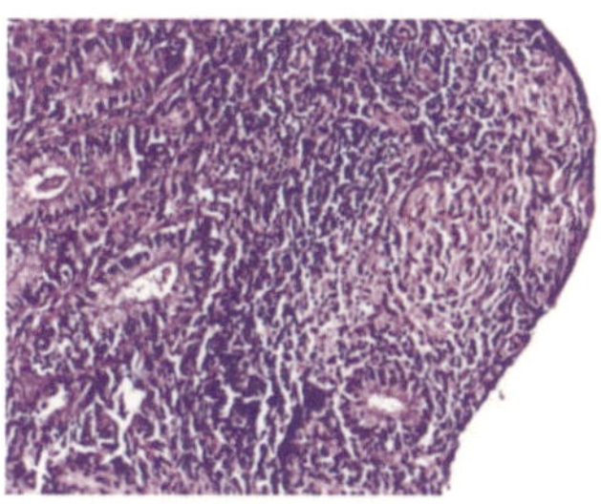

Figure 9.
Patient M.S.A., female, born in 1968. She has been ill since 2017; in 2018, the diagnosis of ulcerative colitis was verified, with total damage to the colon mucosa. (a) Data from endoscopic examination of the colon. Endoscopic conclusion: inflammatory bowel disease, ulcerative colitis, endoscopic remission phase. (b) Data from a pathomorphological study of a biopsy taken from the mucous membrane of the colon. Conclusion of the pathomorphological study: in the biopsy material from the mucous membrane of the colon, the presence of mononuclear cells was revealed against the background of a small number of basal plasma cells; eosinophilic infiltration was detected in the lamina propria (over 35-40 eosinophils 1HPF). The visible picture corresponds to the inactive period of ulcerative colitis (Geboes score 2A.1).

Conclusion: Thus, the increase in the level of ECP in the main group of patients was 27.6%, in this group of patients there were higher indicators of laboratory, endoscopic and morphological activity of IBD; that is, additional determination of eosinophil cationic protein may help identify one of the main reasons for the lack of response in patients with IBD to basic therapy.

8. Is it possible to influence eosinophil activation in IBD?

At diagnosis, patients with IBD are often treated with corticosteroids on a tapering schedule to rapidly improve symptoms (**Table 6**) [11, 86, 87].

Treatment	Influence on eosinophil presence	Influence on fibrostenosis development
Corticosteroids	Prevent eosinophil accumulation and reduce eosinophil chemotaxis and can block other eosinophil factors.	Demonstrated in idiopathic pulmonary fibrosis, systemic sclerosis and retroperitoneal fibrosis: affects wound healing and reduces collagen synthesis.
Anti-α4β7 integrin (Vedolizumab)	Possible ↓ in influx of eosinophils, but inconclusive evidence [80] • Vedolizumab: no effect on eosinophil circulation • Natalizumab: • ↑ in circulating eosinophils • ↓ eosinophil accumulation at site of inflammation	No effects described in literature.
Anti-TNF (infliximab and adalimumab)	No effect described in literature.	Infliximab: suggested to be effective in the early stages of fibrosis development • ↓ in bFGF and VEGF levels in serum • *In vitro* exposure of myofibroblasts, isolated from CD patients, to infliximab: ↓ collagen production. Adalimumab: CREOLE study • CD patients with small bowel strictures: beneficial effect [81]
Anti-IL-12/IL-23 (Ustekinumab)	No effect described in literature.	No effect described in literature.
JAK inhibitor (Tofacitinib)	Effective in several eosinophil related disorders [82–84] • ↓ in eosinophil numbers • ↓ in disease symptoms BAL (Bronchoalveolar lavage) fluid in mice treated with Tofacitinib [85]: • eosinophil presence reduced. • ↓ in [TGF-β] • ↓ myofibroblasts deposited in pulmonary arteries	

Table 6.
Conventional treatment options for IBD patients [11].

Corticosteroids prevent eosinophil accumulation, reduce eosinophil chemotaxis, and may block other eosinophil factors, including eosinophil adhesion in vitro [88, 89]. Corticosteroids are recognized for their antifibrotic properties, achieved through the reduction of collagen synthesis, albeit at the cost of impeding wound healing [90]. This antifibrotic action has been validated across various conditions including idiopathic pulmonary fibrosis, systemic sclerosis, and retroperitoneal fibrosis [91–95]. Nonetheless, prolonged corticosteroid use is discouraged due to its systemic side effects [86].

In recent decades, the treatment landscape for IBD has undergone substantial changes due to the introduction of various biological therapies and small molecules (see **Table 6**). However, the specific impacts of these biologics on eosinophil function, recruitment, and degranulation remain largely unclear. Mucosal addressin cell adhesion molecule 1 (MadCAM-1), located on the endothelial cells lining the blood vessels in the intestinal mucosa, interacts with α4β7 integrin receptors present on the surface of eosinophils. This interaction between α4β7 integrin and MadCAM-1 facilitates the migration of eosinophils into the gastrointestinal tract [86, 87].

Thus, it is expected that anti-α4β7 integrin therapy could influence the recruitment of intestinal eosinophils. However, the evidence in the literature is inconclusive: Bochner BS. reported no effect on eosinophils following vedolizumab treatment [80], whereas natalizumab, a humanized antibody targeting α4β1 and α4β7 integrin approved for systemic sclerosis treatment, resulted in increased circulating eosinophils and decreased eosinophil accumulation at the inflammation site [80]. Non-responders to vedolizumab exhibited a higher mean colonic mucosal eosinophil count at baseline. Further research is warranted to ascertain if this elevated baseline eosinophil count can predict vedolizumab treatment failure [96].

Although the effect of infliximab treatment on the presence and activation status of eosinophils has not been described, it is suggested that infliximab is effective in the early stages of fibrosis. Decreases in serum levels of basic fibroblast growth factor (bFGF) and vascular endothelial growth factor (VEGF) were observed in patients treated with infliximab [11]. These elements are acknowledged for their roles in the development of intestinal fibrosis. Basic fibroblast growth factor (bFGF) fosters the proliferation of fibroblasts, while vascular endothelial growth factor (VEGF) spurs the activation of fibroblasts and the production of extracellular matrix (ECM) components [97]. In the CREOLE investigation, 97 individuals diagnosed with Crohn's disease (CD) and experiencing small bowel strictures underwent treatment with adalimumab. Findings revealed that around two-thirds (63.9%) of CD patients responded positively to adalimumab, with a sustained response rate of 45.7% at a span of 3.8 years. This implies that anti-tumor necrosis factor (TNF) therapy might offer advantages in managing intestinal strictures [81]. Tofacitinib, the initial JAK inhibitor approved for treating moderate to severe UC, has demonstrated effectiveness in various disorders linked to eosinophils, such as hypereosinophilic syndrome, drug hypersensitivity syndrome, and eosinophilic esophagitis [82–84]. In an experimental model of pulmonary eosinophilic vasculitis, the administration of tofacitinib to 8-week-old C57BL/6 mice led to decreased levels of eosinophils in the bronchoalveolar lavage fluid. Furthermore, there was a reduction in the concentration of TGF-β in the lavage fluid, along with a decrease in the deposition of myofibroblasts in the pulmonary arteries. This suggests that tofacitinib may not only affect eosinophil infiltration but also function as an antifibrotic agent [85]. However, tofacitinib did not advance beyond phase II trials in patients with luminal CD [98]. In contrast, the JAK-1 inhibitor filgotinib has displayed promising efficacy in CD, including a notable reduction in VEGF [99, 100].

Because the precise role of eosinophils in inflammation and fibrosis remains unclear, therapies specifically targeting eosinophils are not currently part of the treatment regimen for IBD patients. However, studies in murine colitis models have shown that treatments aimed at eosinophils can reduce inflammation and reshape tissue structure [63]. Targeting CCR3 or eotaxin emerges as a promising therapeutic strategy due to their involvement in eosinophil accumulation. In experimental colitis models, blocking eotaxin-1 with an anti-eotaxin-1 monoclonal antibody (mAb) reduced disease severity and showed efficacy in allergic inflammation models [101]. Inhibition of eotaxin has demonstrated significant benefits in DSS colitis, suggesting its potential for IBD treatment development [102].

Benralizumab, a monoclonal antibody that targets IL-5R and reduces eosinophil levels, has shown effectiveness in asthma patients [103]. A similar antibody has been developed and demonstrated significant improvement in radiation-induced intestinal fibrosis in mice, suggesting its potential as a treatment option for certain inflammatory bowel disease patients [58].

Targeting the ST2/IL-33 pathway could offer benefits for managing symptoms in IBD patients. Several antibodies that block IL-33 are currently undergoing investigation for treating asthma and chronic obstructive pulmonary disease. However, caution is advised when targeting ST2, as it activates various cell types, including ILC2s, T lymphocytes, mast cells, basophils, and other immune cells, indirectly affecting other pathways [39].

In conclusion, as highlighted earlier, extensive eosinophil infiltration in the colon's lamina propria serves as a key predictor of inadequate response to drug therapy among UC patients. This underscores the critical role of monitoring eosinophil levels in individuals with IBD [13].

9. Conclusion

So, what conclusion can be summarized?

Eosinophils and their associated components are significant factors in various inflammatory and fibrotic conditions, including IBD. Despite the elevation of important molecules responsible for eosinophil activation and recruitment in IBD patients, the precise mechanism by which eosinophils exert their effects remains uncertain. The specific impacts of eosinophil-related proteins like ECP, EPO, EDN, and MBP are still unclear. However, the release of TGF-β, which promotes fibrosis, by eosinophils might contribute to intestinal fibrosis in these patients. Present studies mostly provide descriptive findings rather than establishing a definitive cause-and-effect relationship. Therefore, further investigation is crucial to understand the involvement of eosinophil activation and degranulation in inflammation and fibrosis, especially within the intestine. This could lead to the identification of novel therapeutic approaches for managing IBD by targeting inflammation and fibrosis.

And answering the previously asked question: Eosinophilic inflammation in inflammatory bowel diseases – the conductor or the "first" violin, so far the answer is the same: both the conductor and the "first" violin, or, for now, a "one-man show".

Author details

Gulustan H. Babayeva[1,2*], Hikmet I. Ibrahimli[3], Ferid V. Guliyev[4], Gunay V. Asadova[1,4], Umud R. Mahmudov[5], Rafail H. Hasanov[6], Emin Kh. Verdiyev[7], Jamal S. Musayev[8], Aychin I. Hasanova[1], Rashad A. Hasanov[1,9], Nargiz E. Afandiyeva[4], Namig O. Isgandarov[10] and Tunzala A. Maharramova[1,4]

1 Department of Therapy, Azerbaijan State Advanced Training Institute for Doctors Named after A. Alıyev, Baku, Azerbaijan

2 Memorial Hospital, Baku, Azerbaijan

3 Department of Health Organization, Azerbaijan State Advanced Training Institute for Doctors Named after A. Alıyev, Baku, Azerbaijan

4 Department of Invasive Diagnosis and Treatment, National Centre of Oncology, Baku, Azerbaijan

5 Department of Gastroenterology and Endoscopy, Modern Hospital, Baku, Azerbaijan

6 Department of Gastroenterology and Endoscopy, Diaqnoz Medical Center, Baku, Azerbaijan

7 Department of Gastroenterology and Endoscopy, Central Hospital, Baku, Azerbaijan

8 Pathomorphology Department, Baku Pathology Center, Baku, Azerbaijan

9 Department of Gastroenterology and Endoscopy, German Hospital, Baku, Azerbaijan

10 Laboratory Department, Memorial Hospital, Baku, Azerbaijan

*Address all correspondence to: ghbabayeva@gmail.com

References

[1] De Souza HSP, Fiocchi C. Immunopathogenesis of IBD: Current state of the art. Nature Reviews. Gastroenterology & Hepatology. 2016;**13**:13-27. DOI: 10.1038/nrgastro.2015.186

[2] Mirkov MU, Verstockt B, Cleynen I. Genetics of inflammatory bowel disease: Beyond NOD2. Lancet. 2017;**2**:224-234. DOI: 10.1016/S2468-1253(16)30111-X

[3] Zhang M, Sun K, Wu Y, Yang Y, Tso P, Wu Z. Interactions between intestinal microbiota and host immune response in inflammatory bowel disease. Frontiers in Immunology. 2017;**8**:942. DOI: 10.3389 / fimmu. 2017.00942

[4] Coskun M. Intestinal epithelium in inflammatory bowel disease. Frontiers in Medicine. 2014;**1**:24. DOI: 10.3389 / fmed.2014.00024

[5] Rieder F, Fiocchi C, Rogler G. Mechanisms, management, and treatment of fibrosis in patients with inflammatory bowel diseases. Gastroenterology. 2017;**152**:340-350. DOI: 10.1053/j.gastro.2016.09.047

[6] Henderson NC, Rieder F, Wynn TA. Fibrosis: From mechanisms to medicines. Nature. 2020;**587**:555-566. DOI: 10.1038/s41586-020-2938-9

[7] Herrera J, Henke CA, Bitterman PB, Herrera J, Henke CA, Bitterman PB. Extracellular matrix as a driver of progressive fibrosis. The Journal of Clinical Investigation. 2018;**128**:45-53. DOI: 10.1172/JCI93557

[8] Shah K, Ignacio A, McCoy KD, Harris NL. The emerging roles of eosinophils in mucosal homeostasis. Mucosal Immunology. 2020;**13**:574-583. DOI: 10.1038/s41385-020-0281-y

[9] Uhlig HH, Powrie F. Translating immunology into therapeutic concepts for inflammatory bowel disease. Annual Review of Immunology. 2018;**36**:755-781. DOI: 10.1146/annurev-immunol-042617-053055

[10] Filippone RT, Sahakian L, Apostolopoulos V, Nurgali K. Eosinophils in inflammatory bowel disease. Inflammatory Bowel Diseases. 2019;**25**:1140-1151. DOI: 10.1093/ibd/izz024

[11] Jacobs I, Ceulemans M, Wauters L, Breynaert C, Vermeire S, Verstockt B, et al. Role of eosinophils in intestinal inflammation and fibrosis in inflammatory bowel disease: An overlooked villain? Frontiers in Immunology. 2021;**12**:754413. DOI: 10.3389/fimmu.2021.754413

[12] Canavese G, Villanacci V, Antonelli E, Cadei M, Sapino A, Rocca R, et al. Eosinophilia – Associated basal plasmacytosis: An early and sensitive histologic feature of inflammatory bowel disease. APMIS. 2017;**125**:179-183. DOI: 10.1111/apm.12639

[13] Zezos P, Patsiaoura K, Nakos A, Mpoumponaris A, Vassiliadis T, Giouleme O, et al. Severe eosinophilic infiltration in colonic biopsies predicts patients with ulcerative colitis not responding to medical therapy. Colorectal Disease. 2014;**16**:O420-O430. DOI: 10.1111/codi.12725

[14] Runge TM, Dellon ES. Do we know what causes eosinophilic esophagitis? A mechanistic update. Current Gastroenterology Reports.

2015;**176**:139-148. DOI: 10.1007/s11894-015-0458-9

[15] Johnston LK, Bryce PJ. Understanding interleukin 33 and its roles in eosinophil development. Frontiers in Medicine. 2017;**4**:51. DOI: 10.3389/fmed.2017.00051

[16] Weller PF, Spencer LA. Functions of tissue-resident eosinophils. Nature Reviews. Immunology. 2017;**17**:746-760. DOI: 10.1038/nri.2017.95

[17] McBrien CN, Menzies-Gow A. The biology of eosinophils and their role in asthma. Frontiers in Medicine. 2017;**4**:93. DOI: 10.3389/fmed.2017.00093

[18] Al-Haddad S, Riddell RH. The role of eosinophils in inflammatory bowel disease. Gut. 2005;**54**:1674-1675. DOI: 10.1136/gut.2005.072595

[19] Ohta K, Nagase H, Suzukawa M, Ohta S. Antibody therapy for the Management of Severe Asthma with Eosinophilic Inflammation. International Immunology. 2017;**29**:337-343. DOI: 10.1093/intimm/ dxx045

[20] Mendez-Enriquez E, García-Zepeda EA. The multiple faces of CCL13 in immunity and inflammation. Inflammopharmacology. 2013;**21**:397-406. DOI: 10.1007/s10787-013-0177-5

[21] Samitas K, Rådinger M, Bossios A. Current update on eosinophilic lung diseases and anti-IL-5 treatment. Recent Patents on Anti-Infective Drug Discovery. 2011;**6**:189-205. DOI: 10.2174/157489111796887855

[22] Soman KV, Stafford SJ, Pazdrak K, Wu Z, Luo X, White WI, et al. Activation of human peripheral blood eosinophils by cytokines in a comparative time-course proteomic/Phosphoproteomic study. Journal of Proteome Research. 2017;**16**:2663-2679. DOI: 10.1021/acs.jproteome.6b00367

[23] Lampinen M, Backman M, Winqvist O, Rorsman F, Rönnblom A, Sangfelt P, et al. Different regulation of eosinophil activity in Crohn's disease compared with ulcerative colitis. Journal of Leukocyte Biology. 2008;**84**:1392-1399. DOI: 10.1189/jlb.0807513

[24] Paul WE. History of Interleukin-4. Cytokine. 2015;**176**:139-148. DOI: 10.1016/j.physbeh.2017.03. 040

[25] Sokol CL, Barton GM, Farr AG, Medzhitov R. A mechanism for the initiation of allergen-induced T helper type 2 responses. Nature Immunology. 2008;**9**:310-318. DOI: 10.1038/ni1558

[26] Giuffrida P, Caprioli F, Facciotti F, Di Sabatino A. The role of Interleukin-13 in chronic inflammatory intestinal disorders. Autoimmunity Reviews. 2019;**18**:549-555. DOI: 10.1016/j.autrev.2019.03.012

[27] Reichman H, Moshkovits I, Itan M, Pasmanik-Chor M, Vogl T, Roth J, et al. Transcriptome profiling of mouse colonic eosinophils reveals a key role for eosinophils in the induction of s100a8 and s100a9 in mucosal healing. Scientific Reports. 2017;7:7117. DOI: 10.1038/s41598-017-07738-z

[28] Griseri T, Arnold IC, Pearson C, Krausgruber T, Schiering C, Franchini F, et al. Granulocyte macrophage Colony-stimulating factor-activated eosinophils promote Interleukin-23 driven chronic colitis. Immunity. 2015;**43**:187-199. DOI: 10.1016/j.immuni.2015.07.008

[29] Kasaian MT, Page KM, Fish S, Brennan A, Cook TA, Moreira K, et al. Therapeutic activity of an Interleukin-4/Interleukin-13 dual antagonist on oxazolone-induced colitis in mice.

Immunology. 2014;**143**:416-427. DOI: 10.1111/imm.12319

[30] Smith SG, Chen R, Kjarsgaard M, Huang C, Oliveria JP, O'Byrne PM, et al. Increased numbers of activated group 2 innate lymphoid cells in the Airways of Patients with Severe Asthma and Persistent Airway Eosinophilia. The Journal of Allergy and Clinical Immunology. 2016;**137**:75-86. DOI: 10.1016/j.jaci.2015.05.037

[31] Ebbo M, Crinier A, Vély F, Vivier E. Innate lymphoid cells: Major players in inflammatory diseases. Nature Reviews. Immunology. 2017;**17**:665-678. DOI: 10.1038/nri.2017.86

[32] Fulkerson PC, Rothenberg ME. Targeting eosinophils in allergy, inflammation and beyond. Nature Reviews. Drug Discovery. 2013;**12**:117-129. DOI: 10.1038/nrd3838

[33] Pelaia C, Paoletti G, Puggioni F, Racca F, Pelaia G, Canonica GW, et al. Interleukin-5 in the pathophysiology of severe asthma. Frontiers in Physiology. 2019;**10**:1514. DOI: 10.3389/fphys.2019.01514

[34] Sugimoto K, Fujita S, Miyazu T, Ishida N, Tani S, Yamade M, et al. Improvement in ulcerative colitis by Administration of Benralizumab for comorbid refractory bronchial asthma: A novel clinical observation. Inflammatory Bowel Diseases. 2021;**27**:E3-E4. DOI: 10.1093/ibd/izaa225

[35] Verstockt B, Perrier C, De Hertogh G, Cremer J, Creyns B, Van Assche G, et al. Effects of epithelial IL-13rα2 expression in inflammatory bowel disease. Frontiers in Immunology. 2018;**9**:2983. DOI: 10.3389/fimmu.2018.02983

[36] Karmele EP, Pasricha TS, Ramalingam TR, Thompson RW, Knilans KJ, Hegen M, et al. Anti-IL-13Ra2 therapy promotes recovery in a murine model of inflammatory bowel disease. Mucosal Immunology. 2019;**12**:1174-1186. DOI: 10.1038/s41385-019-0189-6

[37] Verstockt B, Verstockt S, Creyns B, Tops S, Van Assche G, Gils A, et al. Mucosal IL13RA2 expression predicts nonresponse to anti-TNF therapy in Crohn's disease. Alimentary Pharmacology & Therapeutics. 2019;**49**:572-581. DOI: 10.1111/apt.15126

[38] Reinisch W, Panés J, Khurana S, Toth G, Hua F, Comer GM, et al. Anrukinzumab, an anti-interleukin 13 monoclonal antibody, in active UC: Efficacy and safety from a phase IIa randomised multicentre study. Gut. 2015;**64**:894-900. DOI: 10.1136/gutjnl-2014-308337

[39] Griesenauer B, Paczesny S. The ST2/IL-33 Axis in immune cells during inflammatory diseases. Frontiers in Immunology. 2017;**8**:475. DOI: 10.3389/fimmu.2017.00475

[40] Jonckheere AC, Bullens DMA, Seys SF. Innate lymphoid cells in asthma: Pathophysiological insights from murine models to human asthma phenotypes. Current Opinion in Allergy and Clinical Immunology. 2019;**19**:53-60. DOI: 10.1097/ACI.0000000000000497

[41] Lampinen M, Fredricsson A, Vessby J, Martinez JF, Wanders A, Rorsman F, et al. Downregulated eosinophil activity in ulcerative colitis with concomitant primary sclerosing cholangitis. Journal of Leukocyte Biology. 2018;**104**:173-183. DOI: 10.1002/JLB.3MA0517-175R

[42] Schmitz J, Owyang A, Oldham E, Song Y, Murphy E, McClanahan TK, et al. IL-33, an Interleukin-1-like

cytokine that signals via the IL-1 receptor- related protein ST2 and induces T helper type 2-associated cytokines. Immunity. 2005;**23**:479-490. DOI: 10.1016/j.immuni.2005.09.015

[43] De Salvo C, Wang XM, Pastorelli L, Mattioli B, Omenetti S, Buela KA, et al. IL-33 drives eosinophil infiltration and pathogenic type 2 helper T-cell immune responses leading to chronic experimental ileitis. The American Journal of Pathology. 2016;**186**:885-898. DOI: 10.1016/j.ajpath.2015.11.028

[44] Ihara S, Hirata Y, Koike K. TGF-β in inflammatory bowel disease: A key regulator of immune cells, epithelium, and the intestinal microbiota. Journal of Gastroenterology. 2017;**52**:777-787. DOI: 10.1007/s00535-017-1350-1

[45] Diny NL, Rose NR, Čiháková D. Eosinophils in autoimmune diseases. Frontiers in Immunology. 2017;**8**:484. DOI: 10.3389/fimmu.2017.00484

[46] Wędrychowicz A, Tomasik P, Pieczarkowski S, Grzenda-Adamek Z, Kowalska-Duplaga K, Fyderek K. Clinical value of serum eosinophilic cationic protein assessment in children with infflammatory bowel disease. Archives of Medical Science. 2014;**10**:1142-1146. DOI: 10.5114/aoms.2013.34415

[47] Abedin N, Seemann T, Kleinfeld S, Ruehrup J, Röseler S, Trautwein C, et al. Fecal eosinophil cationic protein is a diagnostic and predictive biomarker in young adults with inflammatory bowel disease. Journal of Clinical Medicine. 2019;**8**:2025. DOI: 10.3390/jcm8122025

[48] Kovalszki A, Weller PF. Chapter 24: Eosinophils and eosinophilia. In: Rich R, Fleisher T, Shearer W, Schroeder H, Frew A, Weyand C, editors. Clinical Immunology. London: Elsevier; 2013. pp. 349-361

[49] Woodruff SA, Masterson JC, Fillon S, Robinson ZD, Furuta GT. Role of eosinophils in inflammatory bowel and gastrointestinal diseases. Journal of Pediatric Gastroenterology and Nutrition. 2011;**52**:650-661. DOI: 10.1097/MPG.0b013e3182128512

[50] Amcoff K, Cao Y, Zhulina Y, Lampinen M, Halfvarson J, Carlson M. Prognostic significance of faecal eosinophil granule proteins in inflammatory bowel disease. Scandinavian Journal of Gastroenterology. 2019;**54**:1237-1244. DOI: 10.1080/00365521.2019.1670251

[51] Roca M, Varela AR, Donat E, Cano F, Hervas D, Armisen A, et al. Fecal calprotectin and eosinophil-derived neurotoxin in healthy children between 0 and 12 years. Journal of Pediatric Gastroenterology and Nutrition. 2017;**65**:394-398. DOI: 10.1097/MPG.0000000000001542

[52] Plager DA, Loegering DA, Checkel JL, Tang J, Kephart GM, Caffes PL, et al. Major basic protein homolog (MBP2): A specific human eosinophil marker. Journal of Immunology. 2006;**177**:7340-7345. DOI: 10.4049/jimmunol.177.10.7340

[53] Click B, Anderson AM, Koutroubakis IE, Rivers CR, Babichenko D, Machicado JD, et al. Peripheral eosinophilia in patients with inflammatory bowel disease defines an aggressive disease phenotype. The American Journal of Gastroenterology. 2017;**112**:1849-1858. DOI: 10.1038/ajg.2017.402

[54] Barrie A, Mourabet M, Weyant K, Clarke K, Gajendran M, Rivers C, et al. Recurrent blood eosinophilia in ulcerative colitis is associated with severe disease and primary sclerosing cholangitis. Digestive Diseases and

Sciences. 2013;**58**:222-228. DOI: 10.1007/s10620-012-2329-7

[55] Jung Y, Rothenberg ME. Roles and regulation of gastrointestinal eosinophils in immunity and disease. Journal of Immunology. 2014;**193**:999-1005. DOI: 10.4049/jimmunol.1400413

[56] Wick G, Grundtman C, Mayerl C, Wimpissinger TF, Feichtinger J, Zelger B, et al. The immunology of fibrosis. Annual Review of Immunology. 2013;**31**:107-135. DOI: 10.1146/annurev-immunol-032712-095937

[57] Speca S, Giusti I, Rieder F, Latella G. Cellular and molecular mechanisms of intestinal fibrosis. World Journal of Gastroenterology. 2012;**18**:3635-3661. DOI: 10.3748/wjg.v18.i28.3635

[58] Takemura N, Kurashima Y, Mori Y, Okada K, Ogino T, Osawa H, et al. Eosinophil depletion suppresses radiation-induced small intestinal fibrosis. Science Translational Medicine. 2018;**10**:333. DOI: 10.1126/scitranslmed.aan0333

[59] Hur GY, Broide DH. Genes and pathways regulating decline in lung function and airway Remodeling in asthma. Allergy, Asthma & Immunology Research. 2019;**11**:604-621. DOI: 10.4168/aair.2019. 11.5.604

[60] Passalacqua G, Mincarini M, Colombo D, Troisi G, Ferrari M, Bagnasco D, et al. IL-13 and idiopathic pulmonary fibrosis: Possible links and new therapeutic strategies. Pulmonary Pharmacology & Therapeutics. 2017;**45**:95-100. DOI: 10.1016/j.pupt.2017.05.007

[61] Burrello C, Garavaglia F, Cribiù FM, Ercoli G, Lopez G, Troisi J, et al. Therapeutic faecal microbiota transplantation controls intestinal inflammation through IL10 secretion by immune cells. Nature Communications. 2018;**9**(1):5184. DOI: 10.1038/s41467-018-07359-8

[62] Fichtner-Feigl S, Kesselring R, Martin M, Obermeier F, Ruemmele P, Kitani A, et al. IL-13 orchestrates resolution of chronic intestinal inflammation *via* phosphorylation of glycogen synthase kinase-3β. Journal of Immunology. 2014;**192**:3969-3980. DOI: 10.4049/jimmunol.1301072

[63] Masterson JC, Capocelli KE, Hosford L, Biette K, McNamee EN, De Zoeten EF, et al. Eosinophils and IL-33 perpetuate chronic inflammation and fibrosis in a Pediatric population with Stricturing Crohn's ileitis. Inflammatory Bowel Diseases. 2015;**21**:2429-2440. DOI: 10.1097/MIB. 0000000000000512

[64] Dewidar B, Soukupova J, Fabregat I, Dooley S. TGF-β in hepatic stellate cell activation and liver fibrogenesis: Updated. Current Pathobiology Reports. 2019;**3**:291-305. DOI: 10.1007/s40139-015-0089-8

[65] Bystrom J, Amin K, Bishop-Bailey D. Analysing the eosinophil cationic protein – A clue to the function of the eosinophil granulocyte. Respiratory Research. 2011;**12**:10. DOI: 10.1186/1465-9921-12-10

[66] Choi Y, Le Pham D, Lee DH, Lee SH, Kim SH, Park HS. Biological function of eosinophil extracellular traps in patients with severe eosinophilic asthma. Experimental & Molecular Medicine. 2018;**50**(8):1-8. DOI: 10.1038/s12276-018-0136-8

[67] Sutherland DB, Fagarasan S. Gut reactions: Eosinophils add another string to their Bow. Immunity. 2014;**40**:455-457. DOI: 10.1016/j.immuni.2014.04.003

[68] Gurtner A, Gonzalez-Perez I, Arnold IC. Intestinal eosinophils, homeostasis and response to bacterial intrusion. Seminars in Immunopathology. 2021;**43**:295-306. DOI: 10.1007/s00281-021-00856-x

[69] Okpara N, Aswad B, Baffy G. Eosinophilic colitis. World Journal of Gastroenterology. 2009;**15**(24):2975-2979

[70] Alfadda, A. A. Eosinophilic colitis: An update on pathophysiology and treatment M. A. Storr, E. A. Shaffer British Medical Bulletin. 2011. 100. 59-72

[71] Alfadda, A. A. Eosinophilic colitis: Epidemiology, clinical features, and current management M. A. Storr, E. A. Shaffer Therapeutic Advances in Gastroenterology. 2011. 4, 5. P. 301-309

[72] Mehta, P. Eosinophils in gastrointestinal disorders: Eosinophilic gastrointestinal diseases, celiac disease, inflammatory bowel diseases, and parasitic infections, G. T. Furuta Immunology and Allergy Clinics of North America. 2015. 35, 3. 413-437

[73] Bates AW. Diagnosing eosinophilic colitis: Histopathological pattern or nosological entity? Scientifica (Cairo). 2012;**2012**:682576

[74] Gonsalves N. Food allergies and eosinophilic gastrointestinal illness. Gastroenterology Clinics of North America. 2007;**36**(1):75-91

[75] Schäppi MG et al. Eosinophilic myenteric ganglionitis is associated with functional intestinal obstruction. Gut. 2003;**52**(5):752-755

[76] Feakins R, Nunes PB, Driessen A, Gordon IO, Zidar N, Baldin P, et al. Definitions of histological abnormalities in inflammatory bowel disease: An ECCO position paper. Journal of Crohn's and Colitis. 2024;**18**(2):175-191. DOI: 10.1093/ecco-jcc/jjad142

[77] Matsushita T, Maruyama R, Ishikawa N, et al. The number and distribution of eosinophils in the adult human gastrointestinal tract: A study and comparison of racial and environmental factors. The American Journal of Surgical Pathology. 2015;**39**:521-527

[78] Turner KO, Sinkre RA, Neumann WL, Genta RM. Primary colonic eosinophilia and eosinophilic colitis in adults. The American Journal of Surgical Pathology. 2017;**41**:225-233

[79] Schumacher G, Kollberg B, Sandstedt B. A prospective study of first attacks of inflammatory bowel disease and infectious colitis. Histologic course during the 1st year after presentation. Scandinavian Journal of Gastroenterology. 1994;**29**:318-332

[80] Bochner BS. Novel therapies for eosinophilic disorders. Immunology and Allergy Clinics of North America. 2015;**35**(3):577-598. DOI: 10.1016/j.iac.2015.05.007

[81] Bouhnik Y, Carbonnel F, Laharie D, Stefanescu C, Hébuterne X, Abitbol V, et al. Efficacy of adalimumab in patients with Crohn's disease and symptomatic small bowel stricture: A multicentre, prospective, observational cohort (CREOLE) study. Gut. 2018;**67**:53-60. DOI: 10.1136/gutjnl-2016-312581

[82] Damsky WE, Vesely MD, Lee AI, Choi J, Meyer AC, Chen M, et al. Drug-induced hypersensitivity syndrome with myocardial involvement treated with tofacitinib. JAAD Case Reports. 2019;**5**:1018-1026. DOI: 10.1016/j.jdcr.2019.07.004

[83] King B, Lee AI, Choi J. Treatment of Hypereosinophilic syndrome with

cutaneous involvement with the JAK inhibitors tofacitinib and Ruxolitinib. Physiology & Behavior. 2017;**176**:139-148. DOI: 10.1016/j.physbeh. 2017.03.040

[84] Mendoza Alvarez LB, Liu X, Glover S. Treatment-resistant eosinophilic oesophagitis successfully managed with tofacitinib. BML Case Reports. 2019;**12**:10-12. DOI: 10.1136/ bcr-2019-232558

[85] Matsumoto A, Sasaki N, Nagashima H, Akiyama M, Niisato M, Yamauchi K, et al. Tofacitinib suppressed Remodeling of pulmonary eosinophilic Vasculitis in a murine model. Translational Science Journal. 2019;**6**:1-7. DOI: 10.15761/JTS.1000355

[86] Torres J, Bonovas S, Doherty G, Kucharzik T, Gisbert JP, Raine T, et al. ECCO guidelines on therapeutics in Crohn's disease: Medical treatment. Journal of Crohn's and Colitis. 2020;**14**:4-22. DOI: 10.1093/ecco-jcc/jjz180

[87] Harbord M, Eliakim R, Bettenworth D, Karmiris K, Katsanos K, Kopylov U, et al. Third European evidence-based consensus on diagnosis and Management of Ulcerative Colitis. Part 2: Current management. Journal of Crohn's and Colitis. 2017;**11**:769-784. DOI: 10.1093/ecco-jcc/jjx009

[88] Altman LC, Hill JS, Hairfield WM, Mullarkey MF. Effects of corticosteroids on eosinophil chemotaxis and adherence. The Journal of Clinical Investigation. 1981;**67**:28-36. DOI: 10.1172/JCI110024

[89] Loymans RJB, Gemperli A, Cohen J, Rubinstein SM, Sterk PJ, Reddel HK, et al. Comparative effectiveness of long term drug treatment strategies to prevent asthma exacerbations: Network meta-analysis. BMJ. 2014;**348**:1-16. DOI: 10.1136/bmj.g3009

[90] Oikarinen AI, Vuorio EI, Zaragoza EJ, Palotie A, Mon-Li C, Uitto J. Modulation of collagen metabolism by glucocorticoids. Biochemical Pharmacology. 1988;**37**:1451-1462. DOI: 10.1016/0006-2952(88) 90006-8

[91] Vaglio A, Palmisano A, Corradi D, Salvarani C, Buzio C. Retroperitoneal fibrosis: Evolving concepts. Rheumatic Diseases Clinics of North America. 2007;**33**:803-817. DOI: 10.1016/j. rdc.2007.07.013

[92] Vaglio A, Maritati F. Idiopathic retroperitoneal fibrosis. Journal of the American Society of Nephrology. 2016;**27**:1880-1889. DOI: 10.1681/ ASN.2015101110

[93] Badea I, Taylor M, Rosenberg A, Foldvari M. Pathogenesis and therapeutic approaches for improved topical treatment in localized scleroderma and systemic sclerosis. Rheumatology. 2009;**48**:213-221. DOI: 10.1093/ rheumatology/ken405

[94] Peikert T, Daniels CE, Beebe TJ, Meyer KC, Ryu JH. Assessment of current practice in the diagnosis and therapy of idiopathic pulmonary fibrosis. Respiratory Medicine. 2008;**102**:1342-1348. DOI: 10.1016/j.rmed. 2008.03.018

[95] Rogliani P, Mura M, Assunta Porretta M, Saltini C. New perspectives in the treatment of idiopathic pulmonary fibrosis. Therapeutic Advances in Respiratory Disease. 2008;**2**:75-93. DOI: 10.1177/1753465808089363

[96] Kim EM, Randall C, Betancourt R, Keene S, Lilly A, Fowler M, et al. Mucosal eosinophilia is an independent predictor of vedolizumab efficacy in inflammatory bowel diseases. Inflammatory Bowel Diseases. 2020;**26**:1232-1238. DOI: 10.1093/ibd/ izz251

[97] Larsson-Callerfelt A-K, Andersson Sjöland A, Hallgren O, Bagher M, Thiman L, Löfdahl C-G, et al. VEGF induces ECM synthesis and fibroblast activity in human lung fibroblasts. The European Respiratory Journal. 2017;**50**:PA1045. DOI: 10.1183/1393003.congress-2017.PA1045

[98] Panés J, Sandborn WJ, Schreiber S, Sands BE, Vermeire S, D'Haens G, et al. Tofacitinib for induction and maintenance therapy of Crohn's disease: Results of two phase IIb randomised placebo-controlled trials. Gut. 2017;**66**:1049-1059. DOI: 10.1136/gutjnl-2016-312735

[99] Vermeire S, Schreiber S, Petryka R, Kuehbacher T, Hebuterne X, Roblin X, et al. Clinical remission in patients with moderate-to-severe Crohn's disease treated with Filgotinib (the FITZROY study): Results from a phase 2, double-blind, randomised, placebo-controlled trial. Lancet. 2017;**389**:266-275. DOI: 10.1016/S0140-6736(16)32537-5

[100] Roblin X, Serone A, Yoon OK, Zhuo L, Grant E, Woo J, et al. Effects of the Janus kinase 1 (JAK1)-selective inhibitor Filgotinib on circulating cytokines and whole-blood genes/pathways of patients with moderately to severely active Crohn's disease (CD). Journal of Crohn's and Colitis. 2018;**14**:S457-S458. DOI: 10.1093/ecco-jcc/jjz203.663

[101] Adar T, Shteingart S, Ben-Ya'acov A, Shitrit AB-G, Livovsky DM, Shmorak S, et al. The importance of intestinal Eotaxin-1 in inflammatory bowel disease: New insights and possible therapeutic implications. Digestive Diseases and Sciences. 2016;**61**:1915-1924. DOI: 10.1007/s10620-016-4047

[102] Adar T, Shteingart S, Livovsky DM, Shitrit ABG, Mahamid BKM. Inhibition of Eotaxin-1 (CCL-11) ameliorates DSS-induced colitis – A novel potential therapeutic approach for inflammatory bowel disease. United European Gastroenterology Journal. 2013;**1**:A135-A587. DOI: 10.1177/2050640613502900

[103] Mukherjee M, Sehmi R, Nair P. Anti-IL5 therapy for asthma and beyond. World Allergy Organization Journal. 2014;7:32. DOI: 10.1186/1939-4551-7-32